ADVANCES IN
Vascular Surgery®

VOLUME 10

ADVANCES IN
Vascular Surgery®

VOLUMES 1 THROUGH 6, 8 AND 9 (OUT OF PRINT)

VOLUME 7

ADVANCES IN
Vascular Surgery®

VOLUME 10

Editor-in-Chief
Anthony D. Whittemore, MD

Chief Medical Officer, Chief, Division of Vascular Surgery, Brigham and
Women's Hospital; Professor of Surgery, Harvard Medical School,
Boston, Massachusetts

Associate Editors
Dennis F. Bandyk, MD

Professor of Surgery; Director, Vascular Surgery Division, University of
South Florida College of Medicine, Tampa

Jack L. Cronenwett, MD

Professor of Surgery, Dartmouth Medical School; Chief, Section of
Vascular Surgery, Dartmouth-Hitchcock Medical Center, Lebanon, New
Hampshire

Norman R. Hertzer, MD

Department of Vascular Surgery, Cleveland Clinic Foundation,
Cleveland, Ohio

Rodney A. White, MD

Professor of Surgery, University of California at Los Angeles School of
Medicine; Chief of Vascular Surgery, Associate Chairman, Department of
Surgery, Harbor-University of California at Los Angeles Medical
Center, Torrance

Mosby

Mosby

Vice President, Continuity Publishing: Glen P. Campbell
Developmental Editor: Beth Martz
Senior Manager, Continuity Production: Idelle L. Winer
Production Editor: Donna Skelton
Composition Specialist: Betty Dockins

Printed in the United States of America
Composition by Thomas Technology Solutions, Inc.
Printing/binding by Sheridan Books, Inc.

Editorial Office:
Elsevier Science
The Curtis Center
Independence Square West
Philadelphia, PA 19106-3399

International Standard Serial Number: 1069-7292
International Standard Book Number: 0-8151-2730-8

Contributors

John A. Adeniyi, MD
Fellow, Vascular Institute, Albany Medical College, Albany, NY

Frank R. Arko, MD
Assistant Professor of Surgery, Director of Endovascular Surgery, Division of Vascular Surgery, Stanford University Hospital, Stanford, Calif

Victor M. Bernhard, MD
Lecturer in Vascular Surgery, University of Chicago, Pritzker School of Medicine, Chicago, Ill

Jose Roberto M. Borromeo, MD
Fellow of Vascular Surgery, Yale University School of Medicine, New Haven, Conn

William Brinkman, MD
Resident in General Surgery, Division of General Vascular Surgery, Emory University School of Medicine, Atlanta, Ga

Elliot L. Chaikof, MD, PhD
Professor of Surgery, Division of General Vascular Surgery, Emory University School of Medicine, Atlanta, Ga

Benjamin B. Chang, MD
Assistant Professor of Surgery, Vascular Institute, Albany Medical College, Albany, NY

Timothy A. M. Chuter, MD
Associate Professor of Surgery, Division of Vascular Surgery, University of California at San Francisco

R. Clement Darling III, MD
Professor of Surgery, Vascular Institute, Albany Medical College, Albany, NY

Yves-Marie Dion, MD, MSc
Professor, Department of Surgery, Laval University and Centre Hospitalier Universitaire de Québec, Hôpital Saint-François d'Assise, Québec, Canada

Yvan Douville, MD, MSc
Professor, Department of Surgery, Laval University and Centre
Hospitalier Universitaire de Québec, Hôpital Saint-François d'Assise,
Québec, Canada

Mark F. Fillinger, MD
Associate Professor of Surgery, Section of Vascular Surgery,
Dartmouth-Hitchcock Medical Center, Lebanon, NH

Kai U. Frerichs, MD
Instructor of Neurosurgery, Departments of Radiology and Neurosurgery,
Brigham and Women's Hospital, Harvard Medical School, Boston,
Mass

Mitchell H. Goldman, MD
Professor and Chairman, Department of Surgery, University of Tennessee
Medical Center, Knoxville

Carlos R. Gracia, MD
Associate Professor, Department of Surgery, University of California, Los
Angeles

Paul B. Kreienberg, MD
Assistant Professor of Surgery, Vascular Institute, Albany Medical
College, Albany, NY

Glenn M. LaMuraglia, MD
Associate Professor of Surgery, Division of Vascular Surgery,
Massachusetts General Hospital, Harvard Medical School, Boston, Mass

Frank W. LoGerfo, MD
William V. McDermott Professor of Surgery, Harvard Medical School,
Chief, Division of Vascular Surgery, Beth Israel Deaconess Medical
Center, Boston, Mass

Manish Mehta, MD, MPH
Assistant Professor of Surgery, Vascular Institute, Albany Medical
College, Albany, NY

Louis M. Messina, MD
Professor and Chief of Vascular Surgery, University of California, San
Francisco; Co-Chair of Department of Surgery, Moffitt Hospital,
San Francisco

Sasan Najibi, MD
Resident in General Vascular Surgery, Division of General Vascular
Surgery, Emory University School of Medicine, Atlanta, Ga

Giuseppe R. Nigri, MD, PhD
Clinical Fellow in Surgery, Department of Surgery, Massachusetts
General Hospital, Harvard Medical School, Boston, Mass

Alexander M. Norbash, MD
Associate Professor of Radiology, Department of Radiology, Departments
of Radiology and Neurosurgery, Brigham and Women's Hospital,
Harvard Medical School, Boston, Mass

Takao Ohki, MD
Associate Professor of Surgery and Chief of Vascular Surgery, Montefiore
Medical Center and the Albert Einstein College of Medicine, New
York, NY

Kathleen J. Ozsvath, MD
Assistant Professor of Surgery, Vascular Institute, Albany Medical
College, Albany, NY

Philip S.K. Paty, MD
Assistant Professor of Surgery, Vascular Institute, Albany Medical
College, Albany, NY

Richard S. Pergolizzi, MD
Instructor of Radiology, Department of Radiology, Brigham and Women's
Hospital, Harvard Medical School, Boston, Mass

Joseph H. Rapp, MD
Professor, Department of Surgery, University of California, San
Francisco; Chief, Vascular Service, Department of Veterans Affairs
Medical Center, San Francisco

Sean P. Roddy, MD
Assistant Professor of Surgery, Vascular Institute, Albany Medical
College, Albany, NY

Dhiraj M. Shah, MD
Professor of Surgery, Vascular Institute, Albany Medical College,
Albany, NY

Bauer E. Sumpio, MD
Professor and Chief of Vascular Surgery, Yale University School of
Medicine, New Haven, Conn

Thomas T. Terramani, MD
Resident in General Vascular Surgery, Division of General Vascular
Surgery, Emory University School of Medicine, Atlanta, Ga

Fabien Thaveau, MD
Fellow, Department of Surgery, Laval University and Centre Hospitalier
Universitaire de Québec, Hôpital Saint-François d'Assise, Québec,
Canada

Carlos H. Timaran, MD
Chief Resident, Department of Surgery, University of Tennessee Medical
Center, Knoxville

Frank J. Veith, MD
Professor of Surgery and Vice President of General Surgery, Montefiore
Medical Center and the Albert Einstein College of Medicine, New
York, NY

Christopher K. Zarins, MD
Chidester Professor of Surgery, Chief, Division of Vascular Surgery,
Stanford University, Stanford, Calif

Contents

Part I

Carotid Artery Disease

CHAPTER 1

Recurrent Carotid Stenosis

Joseph H. Rapp, MD
Professor, Department of Surgery, University of California, San
Francisco; Chief, Vascular Service, Department of Veterans Affairs
Medical Center, San Francisco

Louis M. Messina, MD
Professor and Chief of Vascular Surgery, University of California, San
Francisco; Co-Chair of Department of Surgery, Moffitt Hospital,
San Francisco

THE LESION

With any injury, there is a healing response involving cellular proliferation and the production of a connective tissue matrix. Within
the arterial tree, the initial response to injury includes wall thickening that encroaches on the lumen. Fascinating recent experimental
data suggest that the majority of the cells found in the recurrent lesions, so called "spindle cells," may arise from circulating hematopoietic stem cells drawn to the injured area.[1]

Given the expected response to injury, it is not surprising that
ultrasound studies after carotid endarterectomy indicate that some
thickening resulting from arterial healing is routine. In most cases
this is self-limited, stabilizing or even beginning to regress 6 to 12
months after surgery. In a small number of patients, this process becomes excessive, eventually producing a significant narrowing of
the lumen. The incidence of this excessive response varies among
authors. With routine ultrasound follow-up, the incidence of a 30%
narrowing may be as high as 30%,[2] the incidence of a 50% stenosis
approximately 10% to 15%, and the incidence of a greater than 80%
stenosis approximately 2% to 3%.[3] The routine use of patching and
possibly the eversion endarterectomy technique have been reported
to significantly lower this incidence.

Stoney and String[4] were the first to describe the bimodal distribution of presentation for those patients whose lesions progressed
to require surgical repair. In their series, early lesions presented at a

mean postoperative interval of 9 months, whereas late recurrent stenoses presented at a mean of 5 years after the original operation. Although this has been interpreted as indicating that there are 2 unique pathologic processes involved in recurrent stenosis, it is more likely a continuum, with those lesions presenting within the first year representing a more aggressive proliferative process. Later lesions simply represent a slower variant of the same process, which begins to take on the appearance of primary atherosclerosis. Pathologic review of the specimens at the University of California, San Francisco (UCSF) demonstrated that lesions removed 1 to 6 years after surgery had progressively greater amounts of lipid with fewer areas of spindle cells alone. Later lesions continued this trend, with some being virtually indistinguishable from primary atherosclerosis.

There were 2 variant lesions identified in the UCSF experience that will be important to identify if angioplasty is to be widely applied to these lesions. One is a stenosis resulting not from a proliferative response but from a scarring cicatrix surrounding the carotid artery, and the other is a lesion consisting of a thick layer of thrombus developing in a vessel with a widened diameter. In our judgment, both of these lesions are best treated by replacing the involved portion of the internal carotid.

ETIOLOGY

LOCAL FACTORS

A combination of local and systemic factors may contribute to an exaggerated healing response, resulting in recurrent carotid stenosis. Although not the most common cause, a residual defect at the site of the endarterectomy increases the likelihood of a restenosis. Certainly, anatomic factors such as irregular or nonfixed end points, clamp injuries, and an anterior, rather than full lateral arteriotomy can contribute to a less-than-ideal lumenal surface after endarterectomy. In a prospective study, Reilly et al[3] demonstrated that small lesions (1-2 mm) did not increase wall thickness in follow-up; however, large lesions did contribute to "restenosis." These lesions were most common at the proximal and distal end points. The performance of the surgery must be meticulous, with complete removal of the distal extent of the atheroma and ensuring that the proximal end of the endarterectomy is adherent to the adventitia and is not allowed to "flap" in the arterial flow. Ideally, this is accomplished without stay sutures. The key to a smooth, natural end point is identifying the plaque transition zone from the media to the intima, allowing the surgeon to "feather" the endarterectomy end point.

As the exaggerated healing responsible for recurrent carotid stenosis affects all cardiovascular interventions, a search for the molecular control points of this process has stimulated many researchers to investigate the complex array of growth factors that appear to have a role in the healing/proliferative process. Several of these factors have been found to have a role in the arterial healing response in animals, but as of yet, there has been no evidence that interventions aimed at inhibiting or eliminating these factors have a role in interrupting the healing response in human beings. In contrast, there are intriguing data from coronary stent trials where 2 approaches with antimitotic therapy have shown promise. Short exposure of the stented area to either gamma or beta radiation can reduce the restenosis rate by approximately 50%.[5] Even more impressive results, a 0% restenosis rate, have been achieved by using stents coated with rapamycin, an antiproliferative drug.[6] If these early results are maintained, we may be on the threshold of an exciting breakthrough in controlling the proliferative arterial healing response.

SYSTEMIC FACTORS

The finding that late lesions causing restenosis acquired many of the characteristics of primary atherosclerosis prompted us to examine patients presenting with carotid restenosis for recognized risk factors for atherosclerosis. We compared the lipid profiles of 20 patients requiring surgery within 2 years of the original endarterectomy with 20 patients operated on during the same period who had minimal carotid wall thickening on follow-up. Univariate analysis found elevated low-density lipoprotein (LDL) apolipoprotein B levels and low high-density lipoprotein (HDL) cholesterol were the best predictors of early intimal hyperplasia.[7] Other studies using routine lipid analysis and often including patients with lower degrees of stenosis have not found a correlation of lipid levels with restenosis. Still others have reported associations of smoking and hypertension with restenosis. In arterial injury models in animals, hyperlipidemia, hypertension, and tobacco exposure all promote a hyperproliferative response. Although the traditional risk factors for atherosclerosis may not be present in all patients with restenosis, when these factors are present they should be treated aggressively.

INDICATIONS FOR INTERVENTION

No controlled trials of recurrent carotid stenosis have established the appropriate indications for treatment based on the natural history of the disease. Recommendations for intervention are generally extrapolations from data based on primary lesions. The one exception to this statement is the more conservative recommendations for intervention on early recurrent lesions that by virtue of their smooth contours are believed to have a lower risk of embolic complications.

In patients who are experiencing ipsilateral hemispheric symptoms referable to the recurrent carotid lesion with a greater than 70% stenosis and without other identifiable lesions, the appropriateness of intervention is clear, even in patients with early hyperplastic lesions. In early lesions, if stenosis is less than 70%, the decision to intervene requires serious consideration of alternative embolic sources to prove beyond a reasonable doubt that removing the recurrent stenosis will remove the source of the embolus. For late lesions, as these resemble primary atherosclerosis, it seems reasonable to apply the findings of the North American Symptomatic Carotid Endarterectomy Trial (NASCET) in which removal of lesions causing 50% to 70% stenosis reduced the incidence of stroke.[8]

When the recurrent carotid lesion is asymptomatic for the first 2 years, a conservative approach seems appropriate, with surgery recommended only when the lesion seems to be progressing towards vessel occlusion. For late lesions, we have adopted a more aggressive approach. We recommend continued follow-up for lesions causing stenosis of less than 80%. For those causing a greater than 80% narrowing that persist for all lesions with major irregular surface contours, we recommend reoperative surgery.

WORKUP

Although ultrasound alone may be considered adequate workup for routine carotid stenosis, we recommend a complete visualization of the carotid artery for evaluation of a recurrent lesion. There may be disease both at the proximal and distal end point of the previous endarterectomy (Fig 1). In addition, since the procedure will likely involve a more extensive exposure of the carotid artery than was done at the original procedure, a precise definition of the extent of the lesion is invaluable. We have found that either magnetic resonance angiography (MRA), which includes the entire extracranial and intracranial carotid artery, or conventional carotid angiography are required. If MRA is to be done, markers should be placed on the angle of the jaw to clarify the location of the recurrent lesion relative to this important landmark.

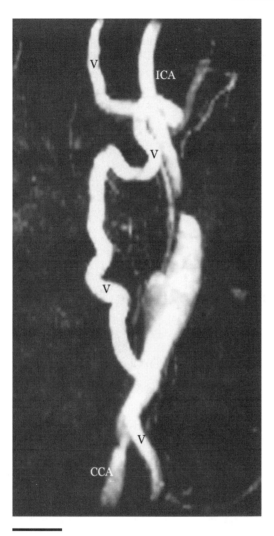

FIGURE 1.

Patient with restenosis at both the distal internal carotid artery *(ICA)* and proximal common carotid artery *(CCA)* end points. He also had an occluded external carotid artery. The vertebral artery *(V)* is also shown in this magnetic resonance angiography (MRA) projection.

INDICATIONS FOR ANGIOPLASTY

Angioplasty has been touted as an alternative to surgery for recurrent carotid lesions. These recommendations come with an almost complete lack of data to support such a fundamental shift in the care of these patients. Although there is certainly a lower risk of cranial nerve injury with angioplasty, there are conflicting data as to its true utility.[9] Angioplasty is certainly an attractive alternative for early recurrent lesions with their theoretically low embolic potential, but even in these lesions there is, as yet, no evidence that angioplasty is comparable to surgery.

For late lesions, angioplasty carries a significant risk of embolization. We have recent data showing that thousands of plaque fragments are released with angioplasty, and the majority of these are not trapped with any of the various filtration devices in current clinical trials.[10] It is not clear that angioplasty offers any real advantage over surgery at this time. Similarly, there are no data to suggest that the indications for intervention would be any different for angioplasty of recurrent lesions than they are for operative repair.

SURGICAL APPROACH

The approach to the recurrent carotid lesion should not simply follow the scar to the carotid artery as has been proposed in other publications. The approach utilizes easily recognized tissue planes to provide wide exposure yet minimize the risk of cranial nerve injury.

EXPOSURE

At the time of the skin incision, we remove the previous scar to improve the cosmetic result. The first landmark after the platysma is the sternocleidomastoid muscle. It is important to expose the anterior border of the sternocleidomastoid along the entire length of the wound and even beyond the wound margin if the recurrent lesion is extensive. Next, the anterior border of the muscle is followed medially and slightly posterior until the internal jugular vein is identified or until the incision is posterior to the carotid pulsation. Then the anterior border of the internal jugular vein is exposed along the entire extent of the wound. Completing the jugular vein exposure before exposing the carotid artery ensures reflection of the ansa hypoglossus and the hypoglossal nerve medially. This maneuver also allows a blunt self-retaining retractor to be placed on the vein to "pin" it and retract it away from the carotid artery. Once this is done, the carotid artery is approached. This is done taking care not to grasp or manipulate the vagus nerve lying between the jugular vein and the artery. Usually, exposure of the carotid artery must extend beyond the previous endarterectomy site. In achieving distal carotid exposure, additional mobility of the hypoglossal nerve can be obtained by ligating the occipital artery. In addition, the digastric muscle can be removed with no disability, although excessive retraction under the mandible can damage the marginal mandibular nerve. Retraction should be directed toward the ear as much as possible to avoid this cosmetically important nerve.

OPERATIVE REPAIR

We generally favor a repeat endarterectomy or myointimectomy in the case of early recurrent lesions, with patch closure of the arteriotomy. Whereas some authors have advised against redo endarterectomy because of difficulty finding the appropriate plane, we have found that it is nearly always possible. An advantage of this technique is that it allows a smaller patch to be securely applied to a well-defined adventitial layer. The artery is always patched with synthetic material. Generally, the goal is to extend the arteriotomy beyond the previous endarterectomy bed.

Replacement of the carotid artery is reserved for patients in whom the extralumenal scarring is so intense that the normal arterial architecture is virtually obliterated, when the carotid artery is patulous, or for the rare patient who has rapidly developed a second recurrence. In general, 6-mm polytetrafluoroethylene (PTFE) is used to replace the vessel, but saphenous vein as long as it is of similar size is equivalent.

After every carotid operation is examined by intraoperative duplex scanning before the patient leaves the operating room.

POSTOPERATIVE TREATMENT

All patients are placed on aspirin therapy postoperatively. In that a single cause of the restenosis has not been identified, we treat all potential contributing factors in the individual patient. Any patient who is still smoking is strongly encouraged to quit. Smokers are most likely to quit during the perioperative period, and this opportunity should not be missed. Patients with elevated cholesterol levels are begun on statin therapy. In addition to their potent lipid-lowering effects, these drugs have anti-inflammatory actions that could be a factor in reducing the response to injury. A low HDL cholesterol level is a risk factor that is difficult to treat unless there is an associated hypertriglyceridemia. Lowering the triglyceride level will raise the HDL cholesterol level and can have a major influence on the overall cardiovascular risk profile. Hypertriglyceridemia is also associated with hyperfibrinogenemia, which along with antiphospholipid antibodies, homocysteine, and possibly the unique lipoprotein Lp(a) can produce a prothrombotic state. This condition should be sought out, especially in young patients with premature disease in whom the more common risk factors are not present.

Our ultrasound follow-up of patients with recurrent carotid stenosis is more intensive than the standard 6-month follow up of patients after primary carotid endarterectomy. We continue to examine the carotid artery every 3 months until the wall thickness is stable and then follow an every 6-month protocol.

OPERATIVE RESULTS

Results from UCSF and other institutions have shown that the stroke rate after reoperative carotid surgery is comparable to that after primary carotid surgery. We reported 116 consecutive operations with a stroke rate of 4.3%.[11] However, in this earlier experience, there were 23 cranial nerve injuries (20%). Our more rigorous anatomic approach to the carotid artery evolved during this experience. While most cranial nerve injuries result from manipulating the nerve and are temporary, these data underscore that a careful approach to the carotid artery is required.

The success of operative repair is excellent. Only 6 patients from our series developed a secondary recurrence. Three of these patients developed early recurrences and were reoperated on at a mean interval of 14 months after their first recurrence. The remaining 3 patients developed recurrences at a mean of 104 months.

RESULTS OF CAROTID ANGIOPLASTY

To date, the number of reports of angioplasty of recurrent lesions is small. Most reports are single-institution experiences and, with a few notable exceptions,[9] the results are encouraging. A recent report of a multicenter registry described a series of 358 patients with a 30-day stroke and mortality rate of 3.7%.[12] The 3-year follow-up of these patients suggested a durable result of this endovascular approach to carotid restenosis. Although these results are encouraging, in our practice we reserve carotid angioplasty for early recurrences that are preocclusive and extend beyond the level of the C2 vertebral body. These are difficult to approach surgically, and the likelihood of peripheral nerve injury is high with these lesions.

REFERENCES

1. Sata M, Saiura A, Kunisato A, et al: Hematopoietic stem cells differentiate into vascular cells that participate in the pathogenesis of atherosclerosis. *Nat Med* 8:403-409, 2002.

2. Civil ID, O'Hara PJ, Hertzer NR, et al: Late patency of the carotid artery after endarterectomy. *J Vasc Surg* 8:79-85, 1988.
3. Reilly LM, Okuhn SP, Rapp JH, et al: Recurrent carotid stenosis: A consequence of local of systemic factors? *J Vasc Surg* 11:448-460, 1990.
4. Stoney RJ, String ST: Recurrent carotid stenosis. *Surgery* 80:705-710, 1976.
5. Waksman R, Raizner AE, Yeung AC, et al: Use of localised intracoronary beta radiation in treatment of in-stent restenosis: The INHIBIT randomised controlled trial. *Lancet* 359:551-557, 2002.
6. Serruys PW, Regar E, Carter AJ: Rapamycin eluting stent: The onset of a new era in interventional cardiology. *Heart* 87:305-307, 2002.
7. Colyvas N, Rapp JH, Phillips NR, et al: Relation of plasma lipid and apoprotein levels to progressive intimal hyperplasia after arterial endarterectomy. *Circulation* 85:1286-1292, 1992.
8. Barnett HJM, Taylor DW, Eliasziw M, et al: Benefit of carotid endarterectomy in patients with symptomatic moderate or severe stenosis. *N Engl J Med* 339:1415-1425, 1998.
9. Leger AR, Neale M, Harris JP: Poor durability of carotid angioplasty and stenting for treatment of recurrent artery stenosis after carotid endarterectomy: An institutional experience. *J Vasc Surg* 33:1008-1014, 2001.
10. Rapp JH, Pan XM, Yu P, et al: Cerebral ischemia and infarction from atheroemboli <100μm in size. *Circulation* 104:II-764, 2001.
11. Bartlett FF, Rapp JH, Goldstone J, et al: Recurrent carotid stenosis: Operative strategy and late results. *J Vasc Surg* 5:452-456, 1987.
12. New G, Roubin GS, Iyer SS, et al: Safety, efficacy, and durability of carotid artery stenting for restenosis following carotid endarterectomy: A multicenter study. *J Endovasc Ther* 7:345-352, 2000.

CHAPTER 2

Treatment of Carotid Artery Disease With Angioplasty and Stenting

Kai U. Frerichs, MD
Instructor of Neurosurgery, Departments of Neurosurgery and Radiology, Brigham and Women's Hospital, Harvard Medical School, Boston, Mass

Richard S. Pergolizzi, MD
Instructor of Radiology, Department of Radiology, Brigham and Women's Hospital, Harvard Medical School, Boston, Mass

Alexander M. Norbash, MD
Associate Professor of Radiology, Department of Radiology, Brigham and Women's Hospital, Harvard Medical School, Boston Mass

Stroke is the third leading cause of death in the United States. The associated cost in human suffering in addition to the loss of productivity and economic loss is unmeasurable. Intra-arterial endovascular therapies for stroke are playing an increasing role in the management of cerebrovascular disease. Early intra-arterial thrombolysis and angioplasty have been found to be effective in improving outcomes in stroke victims within a time window of 6 hours after the onset of symptoms. Endovascular therapies have also found increasing application in stroke prevention, with the use of angioplasty and stent technologies to treat extracranial as well as intracranial carotid and cerebrovascular disease. The purpose of this chapter is to review the current indications and state of the art of carotid stenting and angioplasty. It is important to keep in mind that this technology is very much in flux, with ongoing modifications of its methodology that bear on the comparability with existing treatment options.

HISTORY OF CAROTID ANGIOPLASTY AND STENTING

Carotid angioplasty has been performed since the early 1980s. Lower restenosis rates in the coronary arteries in patients undergoing stent-supported balloon angioplasty versus simple angioplasty alone prompted the first trials of carotid stenting. Several series have been published and have overall shown morbidity and mortality rates that compare favorably to carotid endarterectomy (CEA). Many of the patients undergoing stent placement would not have been eligible for a CEA by North American Symptomatic Carotid Endarterectomy Trial (NASCET) criteria because of their increased risk profile. As this information has been gathered in respect to the technical and clinical efficacy of stenting in a number of cases, a number of trials have now been initiated to explore the direct question of carotid stenting vis-à-vis endarterectomy in patients who would be considered candidates for open surgical treatment. Currently, a large trial is underway directly comparing CEA with stent-supported carotid angioplasty in a randomized controlled setting (CREST).

CAROTID STENTING INDICATIONS

Two broad categories of carotid disease states are currently considered for endovascular stenting: (1) carotid disease states that currently have only suboptimal or challenging open surgical treatment options; and (2) disease states that can be effectively and easily treated with open surgical approaches, and where there is a question of the ultimate clinical utilization of closed endovascular treatment. Examples of the former include carotid dissections, surgically inaccessible lesions, unclampable carotids, and radiation-scarred necks. Examples of the latter and more controversial area initially include rapid postendarterectomy restenosis, and patients with contralateral occlusions.

There has been a gradual evolution during the past 10 years in the range of patients who are considered candidates for carotid stenting. Among the first cases of supra-aortic stenting, carotid stenting was considered a helpful tool in the treatment of postradiation stenoses in patients after neck radiation for head and neck cancers, since the often "woody" fibrotic necks of these patients did not permit easy dissection and exposure of the cervical carotid artery for endarterectomy or repair (Fig 1). Patients with carotid dissections were also early on considered candidates for the procedure, when demonstrating symptoms refractory to conservative nonsurgical management, since the surgical repair of dissections can be chal-

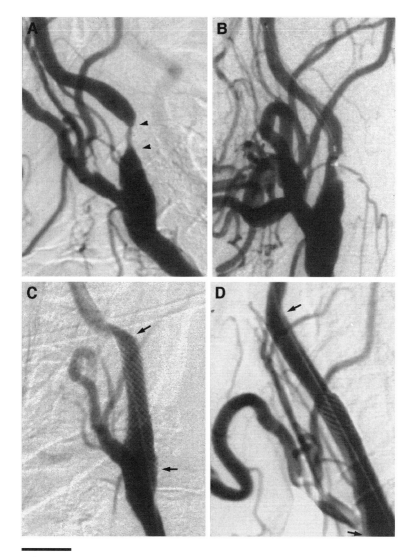

FIGURE 1.

Postradiation stenosis of left carotid artery 13 years after neck radiation for malignancy. A short-segment high-grade stenosis (*arrowheads* in **panel A,** lateral projection digital subtraction angiography) is seen just distal to the carotid bifurcation. After balloon angioplasty **(B)**, a moderate increase in the stenotic lumen is achieved, permitting passage of the stent assembly. The stent is deployed, and poststent balloon angioplasty carried out **(C)** that reconstitutes the normal vessel lumen. A kink at the superior stent margin (inferior and superior stent margins indicated by *arrows* in **panel C**) necessitated the deployment of a second stent distal to and overlapping with the first stent **(D)**. The internal carotid artery distal to the second stent has now resumed the appropriate anatomic course (*arrow* in **panel D**).

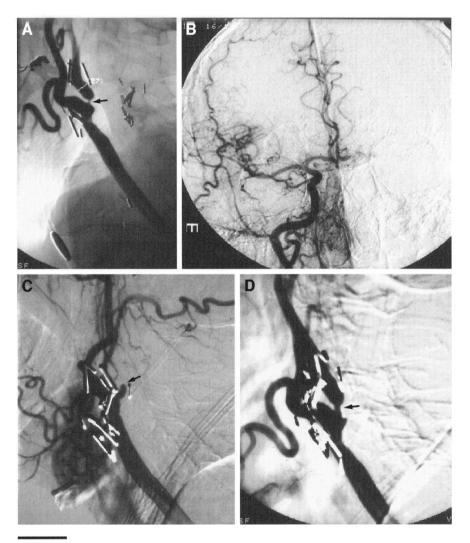

FIGURE 2.

Postendarterectomy stenosis in a patient with blood pressure-dependent symptoms of bilateral hemispheric dysfunction. A high-grade stenosis of the right internal carotid artery is seen just distal to the bifurcation 3 years after carotid endarterectomy (*arrow* in **panel A,** lateral projection digital subtraction angiography [DSA]). This lesion is severely flow limiting, and the intracranial branches fill only sluggishly (**B,** anteroposterior projection DSA). The left internal carotid artery is occluded (**C,** lateral projection DSA). After prestent angioplasty of the right internal carotid lesion, some improvement in the stenotic lumen is achieved (*arrow* in **panel**

(continued)

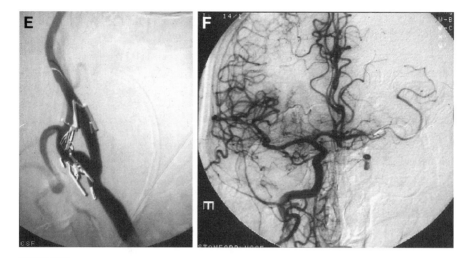

FIGURE 2. (continued)

D). After stent placement, the normal lumen is reconstituted **(E)**, and the intracranial circulation fills more briskly, and crossfilling across the anterior communicating artery into the left middle cerebral artery is now seen **(F)**.

lenging as a result of the complex tissue dissection planes, which may be difficult to identify and tack down operatively. As experience grew, subsequent pathologic states considered amenable to endovascular carotid stenting included fixed high-grade lesions above sites affording ready surgical exposure, and occasional cases where surgical exposure is afforded, although the carotid artery is so densely and homogeneously calcified that a soft cross-clamping site cannot be identified.

More recently, carotid stenting has been implemented in the endovascular treatment of patients who have had rapid restenosis of fixed carotid lesions after prior close-term endarterectomy (Fig 2), as well as for the endovascular treatment of patients with occlusions in the carotid artery contralateral to the site of treatment (Fig 3). Intracranial carotid disease poses a particular management challenge and may, in select cases, be amenable to endovascular stenting (Fig 4). Indications for carotid stenting may further expand if morbidity and mortality and restenosis rates are found to be comparable to the high standards set by the CEA trials.

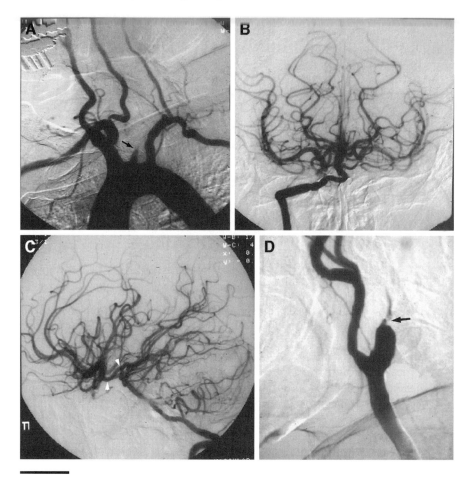

FIGURE 3.

Contralateral occlusion of left common carotid artery close to aortic arch (*arrow* in **panel A,** anteroposterior projection digital subtraction angiography [DSA]) in a patient with right hemispheric transient ischemic attacks. The patient depends on the right vertebral artery to fill the entire intracranial circulation (AP projection DSA in **panel B,** lateral projection DSA in **C**). All 3 territories (anterior, middle, and posterior cerebral arteries) are filled from this single vessel, indicating an anatomically complete and functional circle of Willis. The right internal carotid is subtotally occluded approximately 2 cm distal to the bifurcation (*arrow* in **panel D,** lateral projection DSA). After prestent angioplasty, the luminal diameter of the diseased

(continued)

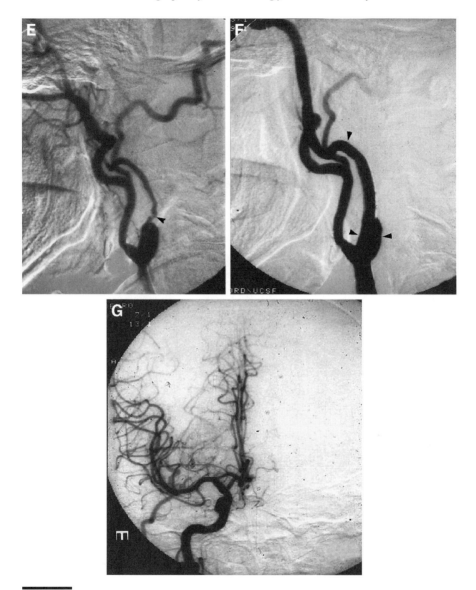

FIGURE 3. (continued)

vessel has slightly increased **(E)**, and after stent placement **(F)**, the normal vessel lumen is reconstituted (upper and lower stent margins outlined by *arrows* in **panel F**). The right middle and anterior cerebral artery territories are now filled from the right internal carotid artery **(G,** anteroposterior projection DSA).

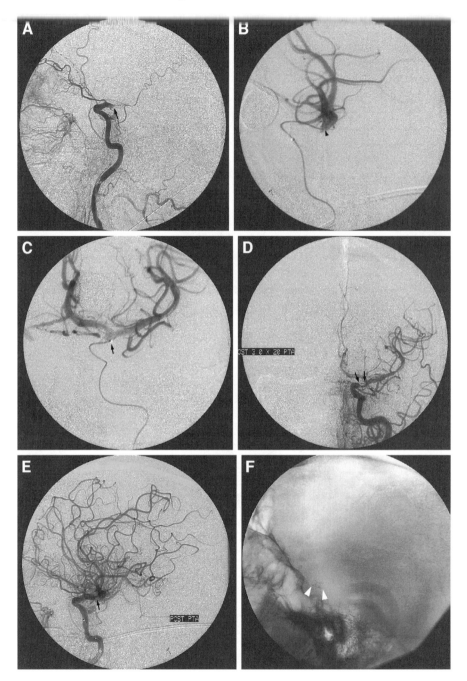

(continued)

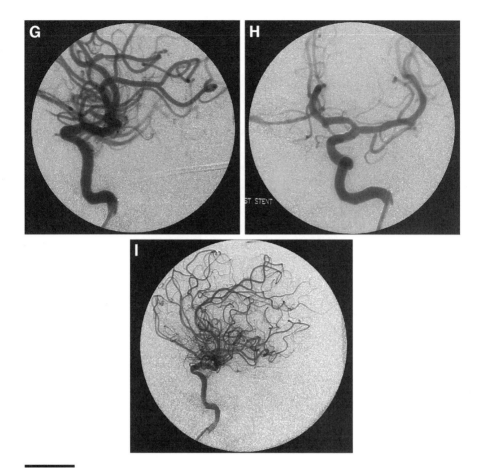

FIGURE 4. (continued)

Intracranial carotid disease in a patient presenting with progressive right hemiplegia, aphasia, and obtundation over 48 hours. The appearance of the cervical carotid artery is normal, but a complete left supraclinoid internal carotid occlusion is seen intracranially distal to the ophthalmic artery (**A,** lateral projection digital subtraction angiography [DSA]). After attempted and unsuccessful intra-arterial thrombolysis with recombinant tissue-type plasminogen activator, a microcatheter is passed blindly through the occluded segment. A superselective injection of contrast through the microcatheter just distal to the occluded supraclinoid carotid segment (*arrows* in **panels B** and **C**) indicates that the distal intracranial branches of the middle and anterior cerebral arteries are patent (**B,** lateral projection, **C,** anteroposterior [AP] projection, high magnification DSA [3×]). Intracranial carotid balloon angioplasty successfully reestablishes flow through the occluded supraclinoid carotid segment (**D,** AP projection, **E,** lateral projection DSA), but with significant residual stenosis (*arrows* in **panels D** and **E**). After stent placement into the stenosed segment (stent in the supraclinoid carotid artery indicated by *white arrowheads* on **panel F**, lateral unsubtracted spot film), the normal vessel lumen is reconstituted (**G,** lateral projection DSA, **H,** AP projection DSA). The final control angiogram (**I,** lateral projection DSA) shows significantly improved intracranial filling. The patient made an excellent recovery and returned to full-time work.

CLINICAL MANAGEMENT

Many variations exist in the clinical management of patients considered for carotid stenting. A variety of technical approaches have been published and produced excellent results. The following section focuses on the protocol used by the interventional neuroradiology service at the Brigham and Women's Hospital.

PREPROCEDURE

All patients undergo evaluation by a multidisciplinary team consisting of the endovascular surgical neuroradiologist, a stroke neurologist, and a neurosurgeon or vascular surgeon. A detailed neurologic examination is performed, and a medical history is taken. A recent non-contrast-enhanced computed tomogram of the head is mandatory to rule out intracranial hemorrhage or large territory stroke. We consider fresh ischemic lesions that are larger than 3 cm^2 on cross-sectional imaging a relative contraindication to stenting and angioplasty because of the increased risk of hemorrhagic conversion after reperfusion. In regards to the triaging algorithm for intervention, some vascular surgeons will perform CEAs based on duplex ultrasound results alone. Although the ultrasound results may reliably indicate the presence of a stenosis, correlation with the actual angiographic findings may be inadequate. The carotid stenting procedure has the obvious advantage of providing a diagnostic carotid cervical and cerebral angiogram as the definitive "gold standard" to assess the degree of stenosis based on NASCET criteria. In addition, this allows detection of associated lesions that may render a cervical carotid revascularization inadequate, such as the presence of a flow-limiting tandem lesion, for example, in the supraclinoid internal carotid artery. Additional clinical workup includes an electrocardiogram and a chest radiograph. Patients that have been selected for carotid stenting electively are commonly placed on antiplatelet regimens preoperatively. Clopidogrel, a strong adenosine diphosphate inhibitor, is used at a dosage of 150 mg twice daily for 2 days before the procedure. In addition, aspirin, 325 mg twice daily, is also started at least two days before the procedure. If the procedure is performed on a more emergent basis precluding oral premedication with clopidogrel, a IIb/IIIa antagonist can be administered intravenously throughout the procedure. These powerful drugs can also be helpful in acute in-stent thrombosis. The level of platelet inhibition should be monitored with the use of an aggregometer. We aim for 70% to 90% inhibition.

INTRAPROCEDURE

Carotid stenting and angioplasty can be performed under local anesthesia, although proponents of general anesthesia believe that general anesthesia adds the benefit of muscle paralysis, and allows the presence of a second person for dedication to the task of sedation and pressure control in the event of agitation or bradycardia. This allows for safer catheter and stent assembly manipulations, especially across the area of stenosis, which is done at our institution with the use of a high-magnification road-mapping technique. Road mapping allows superimposition of a stored image of the opacified blood vessels on a blank fluoroscopic image in real-time, allowing the operator a dynamic opportunity to identify the 2-dimensionally depicted intravascular and extravascular spaces, presuming that there is no interval motion of the patient resulting in misregistration of the fluoroscopic and stored angiographic images. This technique is exquisitely sensitive to image degradation from motion. As described above, an antiplatelet regimen with a IIb/IIIa antagonist is instituted, unless the patient has been preloaded with clopidogrel and aspirin. Some degree of transient bardycardia is anticipated during carotid angioplasty in the area of the carotid sinus. This usually does not occur during stent placement, rather this tends to be during the poststenting "touch-up" angioplasty. Complete asystole is rare. Nevertheless, it is prudent to apply external pacemaker pads. It may even become necessary to place a transvenous cardiac pacemaker. Hypotension can accompany transient bradycardia after angioplasty. Therefore, after induction of general anesthesia or intravenous conscious sedation, a radial arterial catheter is placed for invasive blood pressure monitoring. It is important to communicate closely with the anesthesia team about anticipated blood pressure changes. Intra-arterial access is usually obtained via the femoral route. We use the single-wall puncture technique exclusively to minimize the risk of retroperitoneal hematoma. The arteriotomy puncture site is preclosed with a 6F percutaneous closing suture device (Closer, Perclose, Inc, Redwood City, Calif) that deploys a single suture in the puncture hole. The sutures are secured to the skin on either side of the puncture arteriotomy with Steri-Strips, but not tied. This allows an upsized arterial introducer sheath to a higher French size, which is often necessary to introduce the stent delivery system. This suture can then easily be tied at the end of the procedure for immediate and complete hemostasis. This is particularly useful since the patient is maintained on platelet inhibitors and heparin throughout the procedure. Intravenous heparin is administered after the arterial puncture, and an activated clotting time of 200 to 300 seconds is maintained throughout the procedure. Reversal with protamine is usually not necessary with the use of the percutaneous closure suture device.

A full diagnostic angiogram is carried out initially, which includes size calibration to allow selection of the proper stent diameter and length in regards to the stenosis and native vessel diameters. This step also allows consideration of tool selections, such as the need for initial microwire manipulation and preangioplasty in the event that the stent assembly cannot primarily transgress the stenosis. The diameter of the stent should be oversized by 10% to 20% to avoid the potentially catastrophic complication of stent undersizing and embolization. The length of the stent should comfortably cross the area of narrowing. Lesions close to the carotid bifurcation (<10 mm) should be treated by having the stent extend across the origin of the external carotid artery. This is by far more preferable than having the proximal stent partially protrude into the common carotid artery, potentially providing a thrombogenic edge or fence in a region of high rheologic instability. If possible, a long introducer sheath, such as a Cook shuttle system, is placed just proximal to the lesion for added stability. The stent assembly is then passed coaxially through the sheath and across the lesion. In the event that a Monorail stenting assembly is not used, it is critically important to keep an exchange length guidewire across the lesion at all times with the tip just proximal to the petrous internal carotid artery. This allows over-the-wire exchange of the stent assembly for an angioplasty balloon or other device, if necessary, without having to recross the lesion twice. Repeated crossing of the stenosis should be avoided because of the risk of embolization of plaque debris, dissection, and entanglement within the interstices of the deployed stent. Self-expandable stent systems are the most widely used device for the cervical internal carotid artery, and possess an elastic moment and tendency to expand to a designated size. It is extremely important to keep in mind that just as these stents seek to expand to a predetermined size, so they will also not be balloon expandable to a size greater than that of the "fully expanded" stent. Poststent angioplasty is performed with standard angioplasty balloons. This is the time when the carotid sinus is maximally stimulated. Therefore, 0.5 to 1 mg of atropine may be administered just before angioplasty in the region of the carotid bifurcation. Interestingly, the bradycardia reflex may be found in patients with prior endarterectomies on the same vessel, and even with patch placement as part of endarterectomy reconstruction. After successful stent placement and angioplasty, control angiograms are carried out, including a cerebral angiogram to ascertain whether an embolic event has occurred. Blood pressure control now becomes critical and is maintained at a mean arterial pressure of less than 85 mm Hg to minimize the risk of hyperperfusion syndrome. This is exceedingly important in patients with unilateral occlusions who have undergone repair of high-grade contralateral stenoses with endovascular techniques. The arteriotomy puncture site is closed with a percutaneous closing device (Closer) that provides for safe and immediate hemostasis.

POSTPROCEDURE

A detailed neurologic examination is carried out after stenting and angioplasty. Blood pressure is maintained at a mean arterial pressure of less than 85 mm Hg, and the patient is admitted to the intensive care unit for overnight observation and then discharged the following day. Heparin is stopped at the end of the procedure. Clopidogrel is continued for 6 weeks to minimize the risk of thrombocmbolic complications during the period of reendothelialization of the stent surface, which appears to begin within the first 1 to 2 weeks after stent placement. Aspirin is continued for life. Follow-up is done with carotid duplex ultrasound at 6 months, 1 year, and 2 years after stenting to assess stent patency. If there are any specific questions regarding in-stent restenosis or development of tandem lesions, computed tomographic (CT) angiography is often beneficial in further confirming these findings, or triaging the patient for consideration of a conventional angiogram.

CAROTID STENTING TOOLS

The toolkit for carotid stenting includes the appropriate angiographic machinery, in addition to the catheters and guidewires needed to perform the appropriate carotid artery evaluation for therapy. The toolkit also includes the appropriate platform for stent deployment, in addition to the stent itself, and also whichever carotid embolic protection device is used, if any.

INFRASTRUCTURE

Although carotid stenting can be performed in a wide variety of therapeutic settings, it is advisable to consider certain equipment as the basic minimum equipment necessary to perform a procedure that may result in an intracranial embolic event as a complication. If there is consideration for intravascular treatment of the potential endocranial complications such as thromboembolic disease, then it is necessary to consider performing the procedure either in a subtraction angiographic facility with biplane road-mapping capability, or at a minimum in a single-plane subtraction angiographic room with road-mapping capability. Although it is possible to place a stent angiographically with only fluoroscopy, or with only cine capability for image recording purposes, it is unlikely that the appropriate therapy can be implemented for intracranial thrombolysis in such a setting if a significant embolic complication was to occur.

STENTS

Stents are available in a variety of shapes, sizes, designs, and materials. The variety is probably more a reflection of the imperfections of existing designs rather than the extremely divergent family of applications demanding multiple different tools. Currently, the most tangible limitations have much to do with suboptimal flexibility, the challenge in predictably placing stents with millimeter accuracy in rapidly tapering vessels, and flush with vessel origins. In spite of the dramatic advances that have already been made in the field of Materials Sciences, with more flexible assemblies, more conformable stents, thinner profile catheters, softer tipped catheters, and smaller diameter guidewires, there still are significant limitations in regards to access and stent placement when addressing tortuous circulations, such as patients who have hairpin small-diameter arterial turns at the target site for treatment.

There are two broad families of stents: balloon-expandable stents and self-expanding stents. Balloon-expandable stents are thin-walled metallic tubes that are deformable. They are either manually slip-fitted and crimped on a selected angioplasty balloon, or are available premounted from the vendor on an appropriate range of balloons. Self-expanding stents are "springy" and are contained within a constraining tube. To place them, they are positioned across the desired location to be stented, and then are released from a radially constraining catheter. Because of the design element considerations, there tends to be greater flexibility of the assemblies of balloon-mounted stents, and there also tends to be greater precision of placement with balloon-mounted stents that diametrically expand as the balloon inflates, rather than having the greater foreshortening and occasional slight "sliding" that may occur with the self-expanding stents. The one significant advantage of the self-expanding stents in comparison with the balloon-expandable stents is the natural tendency, or springiness, which confers its most conspicuous advantage when considering positioning in an exposed location such as the cervical carotid artery. Specifically, if a balloon-expandable stent is in a compressible site, such as the carotid bifurcation, then manual compression by an examiner can potentially result in accidental crimping of the stent and resultant vessel occlusion. Alternatively, if there is manual compression of a self-expanding stent, then the natural tendency to return to a baseline shape will permit the stent to "spring" back to a patent contour.

In spite of the design differences in the 2 broad families of stents, it is still often necessary to perform an in-stent angioplasty that encourages the stent to open to the optimal diameter. This poststenting in-stent angioplasty, also known as a "touch-up angioplasty," is necessitated by the need to open the stenosis and stent to a full diameter in a sufficiently forced manner so that the tendency to recontract is overcome.

In preparation for actual stent placement, it is occasionally necessary to perform prestenting angioplasty, so that the stent assembly itself can negotiate a preocclusive or extremely high-grade stenosis. Controversy exists performing prestent angioplasty in patients with adequate clearance for the stent assembly, but in whom stent to wall apposition may be improved by such a maneuver. The controversy lies in the question of risk related to the prestent angioplasty, where there is a hypothetical increased risk of downstream emboli if an additional "unnecessary" angioplasty is performed.

To minimize the risk of downstream emboli, carotid protection devices have been created. The intention of these devices is to either capture and remove emboli from the circulation, or else to redirect the emboli to a clinically "harmless" or less harmful location. The 2 broad families of these protection devices can be considered balloons and filters. The 2 specific types of balloon-based protection devices are occluders to flow and reversers to flow. An occluder to flow can be placed above the site of intervention to create a site of stasis, so that all generated particles enter a cul-de-sac, to be removed before balloon deflation after stent placement. A balloon that is a flow reverser is a device such as a balloon-tipped guiding catheter through which the stent placement is performed. The balloon-tipped guiding catheter is placed in the common carotid artery below the site of stent positioning, and the guiding catheter is connected to a low-pressure circuit that permits a reversal in the suprastent flow so that all created emboli are "aspirated" into the guiding catheter and removed from the body. Clearly, this type of device makes certain demands on the circulation, so that cerebral ischemia is not induced during the intervention, in light of there being not only an occlusion to antegrade flow, but even a reversal to the normal caudocranial carotid flow.

In regards to "filtering" protection devices, 3 specific families of issues have been generated: (1) what is the acceptable filtration size below which emboli are clinically harmless? (2) what is the effectiveness of device-to-wall apposition that allows through vascular filtration? and (3) how easy is it to remove the "sack of emboli" from the craniocerebral circulation, once the entrapment and stenting process is complete?

Covered stents have been created to (1) modify the endoluminal treatment site to decrease the chance of restenosis in the longer term, or decrease the release of variously composed microemboli from the endoluminal territory in the short-term and (2) to create a new endoluminal surface that can exclude from the circulation such pathologic lesions as pseudoaneurysms and dissecting hematomas. The disadvantages of covered stents when compared with conventional stents include the mechanical differences, such as decreased flexibility and increased device deployment friction. Covered stents have hypothetical disadvantages when compared with uncovered stents, such as the amount of surface area on which platelets may adhere.

Microstents, which were designed for coronary applications, have been used to access the intracranial circulation. These devices are sufficiently flexible to allow access to many, but not all, patients' intracranial circulations. They have been used to either address fixed stenoses, or to assist in the creation of a neolumen in patients who have aneurysms that are sufficiently wide-necked that they cannot otherwise hold a coil mass intended to remain outside the parent vessel lumen.

COMPLICATIONS

The 3 major categories of specific stent-related complications are intraprocedural complications, perioperative postprocedural complications, and delayed complications. Intraprocedural complications include thromboembolic complications of stenting, stent mispositioning, and intra-arterial stent loss.

In addition to the specific stent-related complications are the complications associated with angiography itself, including contrast-related complications and puncture site complications. Contrast-related complications include allergic reactions and contrast nephropathy. Puncture site complications include retroperitoneal hematomas, femoroinguinal dissections and occlusions, groin hematomas, and complications related to femoral arteriotomy closure devices and aids.

Regarding the therapy of accidentally created intracranial emboli, it is important to clinically consider the cost-benefit ratio of pursuing the particular embolus. As an example, if the embolus is a macroembolus lodged at the supraclinoid internal carotid bifurcation with occlusion to antegrade flow of the anterior and middle cerebral circulations, then since the natural history is a greater than 90% mortality rate, it is important to pursue the macroembolus with an intention to fragment, lyse, or remove it. Greater analysis is necessary with smaller emboli, which should also be considered in the clinical context. As an example, one would more aggressively pursue branch emboli lodged in eloquent cortex than in noneloquent cortex. Eloquent carotid distribution cortex can be considered Broca and Wernicke's regions, the occipital visual cortex in patients with dominant posterior communicating arteries, and the parietal motor strip.

One of the complications of carotid stenting is that of creating or extending carotid dissections. Nevertheless, it is important to avoid chasing dissections that may extend intracranially or above a readily treatable site, when it becomes a futile exercise. Patients who have occlusions of internal carotid arteries may have an undistinguished clinical presentation if there is sufficient cross-circulation from adjoining cerebral circulations. As such, it is important to consider the patency of the circle of Willis when that information is available, and is a compelling reason to consider making routine preprocedure examinations directed at assessing the circle patency, such as CT angiography or magnetic resonance angiography. When there is a question of functional circulation in the circle of Willis, and if there is operator concern regarding the chances for success, then the operator has to give serious consideration to some type of therapeutic alternative such as extracranial to intracranial bypass procedures, or the operator may need to do more elaborate functional testing such as with a balloon test occlusion with hypotensive challenge.

A number of technical complications are possible with stenting, among which are technically predictable problems such as the placement of a stent with too small a diameter across a site of stenosis, the inability to access the target region with the stent assembly, the inability to deploy the stent completely, and the loss of a stent in a large-diameter parent vessel. It is outside the scope of this chapter to technically discuss how the operator deals with each of these complications; clearly, significant experience with snares, stents, thrombolytics, and intravascular and intracranial catheter-based techniques allows the operator a greater chance of addressing each complication as it is encountered.

Large trials are currently underway or being organized that intend to answer a number of stent-related questions as varied as the direct comparison of carotid stenting with surgical endarterectomy, and the importance of carotid protection devices when compared with unprotected procedures. Each of these procedures includes one of a variety of stents, with dramatic differences in mechanical or biological properties between the stents, between their catheter and stent assemblies, and protection devices.

FUTURE DIRECTIONS IN STENTING

As previously stated, 2 large families of pathologic processes may be considered for intracranial stenting, including fixed stenoses and wide-necked aneurysms. In regards to intracranial fixed stenosis stenting, it is unknown whether the restenosis rate is improved if primary stent placement is performed for a high-grade fixed stenosis, rather than initially performing an intracranial angioplasty to be followed by stenting if the stenosis is refractory to angioplasty alone, or whether there is short-term restenosis on follow-up of the primary angioplasty. In addition, a number of intracranial aneurysms are wide-necked and cannot contain a curative coil mass without the risk of the coil mass sliding out of the aneurysm and at least partially into the parent vessel. To address this tendency of the coil mass to slide out of the wide-necked aneurysm, a stent can be placed to bridge the neck of the wide-necked aneurysm, so that the intra-aneurysmal coil mass is held in place by the stent struts and kept from projecting into the parent vessel.

In regards to intracranial fixed stenoses, there are currently a limited number of absolute cases that demand intracranial angioplasty, and conventional treatment primarily relies on medical therapy such as anticoagulants, with endovascular treatment considered only a treatment method for those cases in which medical treatment is unsuccessful. Nevertheless, retrospective series have already demonstrated a suitably low incidence of complications with the endovascular treatment of intracranial atherosclerotic disease so that investigators are considering and organizing trials to compare the efficacy of traditional conservative medical therapy with that of aggressive and earlier endovascular interventions.

As discussed previously in the section describing the broad categories of stents, covered stents have been created that allow intentional exclusion of aneurysms and pseudoaneurysms from the circulatory path. These stents tend to be much less flexible than noncovered stents; nevertheless, they confer unique advantages to the treatment of broad categories of disease. One problem of intracranial aneurysm therapy with covered stents is the dilemma of keeping essential perforator arteries open while eliminating flow into aneurysm. The perforator vessels of the brain often supply eloquent circulation and are often difficult to visualize even with an operative microscope. In addition, the circle of Willis gives rise to numerous perforator vessels, and as luck would have it, most aneurysms are also located on the circle of Willis. Explorations are directed at identifying the optimal configuration and design of high-coverage density, or fine-mesh stents, which may someday be used in the treatment of intracranial aneurysms. It is hypothesized that by altering the turbulence and inflow pressure into an aneurysm, such as may be accomplished with a fine mesh covering the endovascular aspect of the aneurysm neck, it may not only be possible to encourage thrombosis of the aneurysm, but it may even be possible to allow patency of adjoining organized-flow perforator vessels.

CONCLUSION

Even the most diehard of endovascular proponents must admit that certain patients, such as those with extreme carotid artery elongation and tortuosity with coexisting stenotic disease, are more appropriately treated with open surgery than with endovascular techniques. Similarly, even the most conservative of open surgeons must admit that certain patients, such as those with an intrapetrous stenosis who have crescendo transient ischemic attacks in the face of full anticoagulation, may benefit from endovascular stenting. Somewhere between the acceptance of the 2 extremes lies the most appropriate consensus position for the clinical efficacy of carotid stenting in the therapeutic armamentarium for carotid disease, and lies the true challenge that we face as endovascular and open surgeons seeking the most appropriate treatment algorithms for our patients.

REFERENCES

1. Furlan A, Higashida R, Wechsler L, et al: Intra-arterial prourokinase for acute ischemic stroke. The PROACT II study: A randomized controlled trial. Prolyse in Acute Cerebral Thromboembolism. *JAMA* 282:2003-2011, 1999.
2. Mathur A, Roubin GS, Iyer SS, et al: Predictors of stroke complicating carotid artery stenting. *Circulation* 97:1239-1245, 1998.
3. Mericle RA, Kim SH, Lanzino G, et al: Carotid artery angioplasty and use of stents in high-risk patients with contralateral occlusions. *J Neurosurg* 90:1031-1036, 1999.
4. Chastain HD, Gomez CR, Iyer S, et al: Influence of age upon complications of carotid artery stenting. UAB Neurovascular Angioplasty Team. *J Endovasc Surg* 6:217-222, 1999.
5. Lanzino G, Guterman LR, Hopkins LN: The case for stenting. *Clin Neurosurg* 45:249-255, 1999.

6. Lanzino G, Mericle RA, Lopes DK, et al: Periprocedure transluminal angioplasty and stent placement for recurrent carotid artery stenosis. *J Neurosurg* 90:688-694, 1999.

7. Jordan WD, Schroeder PT, Fisher WS, et al: A comparison of angioplasty with stenting versus endarterectomy for the treatment of carotid artery stenosis. *Ann Vasc Surg* 11:2-8, 1997.

8. Naylor AR, Bolia A, Abbott RJ, et al: Randomized study of carotid angioplasty and stenting versus carotid endarterectomy: A stopped trial. *J Vasc Surg* 28:326-334, 1998.

9. Hobson RW: CREST (Carotid Revascularization Endarterectomy versus Stent Trial): Background, design, and current status. *Semin Vasc Surg* 13:139-143, 2000.

10. Shawl F, Kadro W, Domanski MJ, et al: Safety and efficacy of elective carotid artery stenting in high-risk patients. *J Am Coll Cardiol* 35:1721-1728, 2000.

11. Malek AM, Higashida RT, Phatouros CC, et al: Treatment of posterior circulation ischemia with extracranial percutaneous balloon angioplasty and stent placement. *Stroke* 30:2073-2085, 1999.

12. Bejjani GK, Monsein LH, Laird JR, et al: Treatment of symptomatic cervical carotid dissections with endovascular stents. *Neurosurgery* 44:755-760, 1999.

13. Connors JJ, Seidenwurm D, Wojak JC, et al: Treatment of atherosclerotic disease at the cervical carotid bifurcation: Current status and review of the literature. *AJNR Am J Neuroradiol* 21:444-450, 2000.

14. Phatouros CC, Higashida RT, Malek AM, et al: Carotid artery stent placement for atherosclerotic disease: Rationale, technique, and current status. *Radiology* 217:26-41, 2000.

15. White CJ, Gomez CR, Iyer SS, et al: Carotid stent placement for extracranial carotid artery disease: Current state of the art. *Cathet Cardiovasc Interv* 51:339-346, 2000.

16. Marks MP, Dake MD, Steinberg GK, et al: Stent placement for arterial and venous cerebrovascular disease: Preliminary experience. *Radiology* 191:441-446, 1994.

17. Veith FJ, Amor M, Ohki T, et al: Current status of carotid bifurcation angioplasty and stenting based on a consensus of opinion leaders. *J Vasc Surg* 33:S111-S116, 2001.

18. North American Symptomatic Carotid Endarterectomy Trial Collaborators: Beneficial effect of carotid endarterectomy in symptomatic patients with high-grade carotid stenosis. *N Engl J Med* 325:445-453, 1991.

19. New G, Roubin GS, Iyer SS, et al: Use of the glycoprotein IIb/IIIa inhibitor eptifibatide in a patient undergoing carotid artery stenting. *J Invasive Cardiol* 12:23D-24D, 2000.

20. Tong FC, Cloft HJ, Joseph GJ, et al: Abciximab rescue in acute carotid stent thrombosis. *AJNR Am J Neuroradiol* 21:1750-1752, 2000.

21. Chamberlin JR, Lardi AB, McKeever LS, et al: Use of vascular sealing devices (VasoSeal and Perclose) versus assisted manual compression

(Femostop) in transcatheter coronary interventions requiring abciximab (ReoPro). *Cathet Cardiovasc Interv* 47:143-147, 1999.

22. Cura FA, Kapadia SR, L'Allier PL, et al: Safety of femoral closure devices after percutaneous coronary interventions in the era of glycoprotein IIb/IIIa platelet blockade. *Am J Cardiol* 86:780-782, A789, 2000.

23. Shindo H, Ito H, Yoshioka H, et al: [Electron-microscopic study on the effect of an expandable metallic stent placement in the aortic wall]. *Nippon Igaku Hoshasen Gakkai Zasshi* 52:351-357, 1992.

24. Parodi JC, La Mura R, Ferreira LM, et al: Initial evaluation of carotid angioplasty and stenting with three different cerebral protection devices. *J Vasc Surg* 32:1127-1136, 2000.

25. Martin JB, Pache JC, Treggiari-Venzi M, et al: Role of the distal balloon protection technique in the prevention of cerebral embolic events during carotid stent placement. *Stroke* 32:479-484, 2001.

CHAPTER 3

Simultaneous Bilateral Carotid Endarterectomy

R. Clement Darling III, MD
Professor of Surgery, Vascular Institute, Albany Medical College, Albany, NY

John A. Adeniyi, MD
Fellow, Vascular Institute, Albany Medical College, Albany, NY

Sean P. Roddy, MD
Assistant Professor of Surgery, Vascular Institute, Albany Medical College, Albany, NY

Benjamin B. Chang, MD
Assistant Professor of Surgery, Vascular Institute, Albany Medical College, Albany, NY

Paul B. Kreienberg, MD
Assistant Professor of Surgery, Vascular Institute, Albany Medical College, Albany, NY

Kathleen J. Ozsvath, MD
Assistant Professor of Surgery, Vascular Institute, Albany Medical College, Albany, NY

Philip S.K. Paty, MD
Assistant Professor of Surgery, Vascular Institute, Albany Medical College, Albany, NY

Manish Mehta, MD, MPH
Assistant Professor of Surgery, Vascular Institute, Albany Medical College, Albany, NY

Dhiraj M. Shah, MD
Professor of Surgery, Vascular Institute, Albany Medical College, Albany, NY

Coexistence of symptomatic coronary artery disease and signifi-cant carotid artery stenosis ranges from 3.4% to 22%.[1-6] Coronary artery bypass grafting (CABG) in a patient with an internal carotid artery (ICA) stenosis of more than 50% is associated with a postoperative stroke rate of 6%, which increases to more than 16% when the narrowing exceeds 90%.[3-6] This has led many to advocate a variety of approaches addressing the carotid and the coronary atherosclerotic disease. Options include performing the carotid endarterectomy (CEA) in a separate setting before CABG, performing the CABG first and then the CEA on a subsequent admission, or performing both procedures at the same operation. Thus, patients with such extensive disease requiring CABG present a technical as well as a logistic challenge. Balancing the risk of perioperative stroke during myocardial revascularization with the risk of a significant myocardial event after CEA makes the first 2 options difficult. The goal in this subset of patients is to minimize cerebral ischemic events, myocardial infarctions, or both that often accompany separate sequential operations. To accomplish this in patients with unilateral hemodynamically significant carotid stenosis, we have elected to perform CEA at the same time as CABG. During the last 9 years, we have had a stroke/mortality rate of 4.1% in 563 patients.[7]

An even smaller subset of patients have either symptomatic unilateral or high-grade bilateral carotid stenosis.[8-10] Nunn[11] reported a 58% stroke rate in untreated patients with bilateral carotid stenosis undergoing CABG. When only one of the carotid arteries is addressed at the time of cardiac surgery, Hertzer et al[12] reported a significant number in their series developed strokes in the territory of the contralateral nonoperated but diseased carotid artery. A more recent study documented that patients with bilateral carotid artery disease had a 23% incidence of stroke in the untreated contralateral side.[13] When faced with the dilemma of bilateral carotid disease without significant coronary artery disease, our group has had an evolution in thinking. We initially treated bilateral disease 6 weeks apart in staged procedures. We slowly decreased the time between these surgeries, and now perform them only 1 day apart. Obviously, the potential risks associated with performing bilateral neck dissections only 24 hours apart include vocal cord paralysis resulting in respiratory failure, bilateral hematoma formation with compression on the trachea, swallowing and aspiration issues, a potential increased risk for stroke, the length of surgery, and the theoretic potential for an increase in hyperperfusion injury. As we analyzed our results with decreasing time between procedures, we noticed no change in our morbidity or mortality rates. Currently, our series of bilateral sequential procedures includes 527 patients with a stroke/mortality rate of 1.5%.

The presence of either bilateral or unilateral carotid artery occlusive disease is a risk factor for the development of neurologic injury after cardiac operations in both the early and late perioperative periods. Most reports on this dilemma propose that one address the more critical carotid lesion at the time of CABG and subsequently perform the contralateral CEA after a given period of recuperation. In an attempt to minimize the risk of perioperative stroke in this patient population, we and others have performed bilateral CEA immediately followed by coronary revascularization during the same surgical operation.[14-21] We performed our first simultaneous bilateral CEA and CABG in January 1994, and since then have performed 67 cases. The following is a summary of our experience.

INDICATIONS AND PATIENT SELECTION

All patients with unstable angina scheduled for elective or urgent coronary revascularization who had a history of cerebrovascular disease or had a cervical bruit on auscultation of the neck underwent evaluation of their carotid arteries. At our institution, the preferred screening tool is color-flow duplex ultrasound, using the criteria developed at the University of Washington to determine the presence and degree of carotid stenosis.[22] A recent internal review at our institution of patients evaluated from 1995 to the present comparing color-flow duplex ultrasound with angiography and operative specimens demonstrated a high level of accuracy with the noninvasive technique. Patients with narrowing of 80% or more in one or both carotid arteries are candidates for a combined approach. We obtain a second confirmatory test with either magnetic resonance or contrast arteriography when ultrasound findings are equivocal or suggest the presence of bilateral disease. All patients with confirmed 80% or more stenosis of both carotid arteries were offered bilateral CEA at the same time as their CABG.

OPERATIVE PROCEDURE

Separate teams composed of cardiothoracic and vascular surgeons performed the combined procedures. The carotid artery dissection is performed sequentially before endarterectomy, while the cardiac surgery team harvests the saphenous vein. After both carotid artery bifurcations are exposed, the CEAs are performed sequentially. Our preference is not to use any intraoperative neurologic monitoring, and we do not shunt. After completion of the endarterectomies, the

wounds are left open until the patient is weaned off cardiopulmonary bypass and the anticoagulation is reversed with protamine zinc
sulphate. We preferentially have used the eversion technique for
CEA. The primary advantages of eversion endarterectomy are the
removal of the plaque, visualization of the end point, and expeditious reanastomosis or closure of the arteriotomy. With this technique, reanastomosis of the ICA onto the common carotid artery
(CCA) can be performed more quickly and simply, given the anastomosis is on the larger part of the 2 vessels. In our hands, this has
minimized the risk of closure-related problems (restenosis and
thrombosis) while keeping the ICA cross-clamp time to a minimum.
A brief description of the technique follows.

TECHNICAL DETAILS

Both the CCA and bifurcations are exposed. The patient is systemi-
cally anticoagulated with intravenous heparin, 30 IU per kilogram
of body weight. The ICA, external carotid artery (ECA), and CCA are
clamped on one side. Although circumferential dissection of the

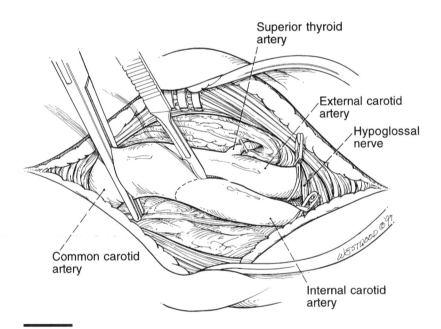

FIGURE 1.

Transection of internal carotid artery. (Copyright 1997, William B. Westwood.)

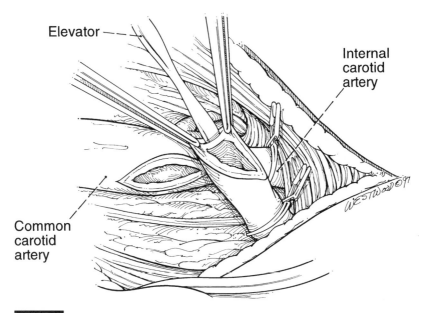

Elevator

Internal carotid artery

Common carotid artery

FIGURE 2.

Elevation of internal carotid plaque. (Copyright 1997, William B. Westwood.)

ICA along its length is a necessary part of eversion endarterectomy, this is probably best completed after division of the artery. Thus, only enough dissection to allow clamping need be performed initially. The end of the plaque may be seen as the transition from the yellowish diseased artery to a normal bluish hue. The clamp should be placed across the normal distal artery, well above the transition zone, as this will make eversion of the artery and examination of the end point in detail easier.

After clamping, the ICA is divided obliquely at the carotid bulb (Fig 1). The actual angle of transection need not be precise but should be in the range of 30° to 60° from the horizontal. After the ICA is divided, upward and lateral traction on the artery will help the operator see the remaining tissue adherent to the artery. This consists of the carotid sinus tissue medially and the looser areolar tissue adherent posteriorly investing the vagus nerve. Dissection directly along the divided artery allows for adequate mobilization while avoiding injury to surrounding structures. Once fully mobilized, the ICA is usually redundant in relation to the CCA.

Removal of the bulk of the ICA plaque is a simple maneuver. The plaque is elevated from the adventitia circumferentially (Fig 2).

Once a reasonable plane is identified, one pair of forceps is used to grasp the plaque, and a second forceps is used to grasp the adventitia. The adventitia is then everted, actually turning inside out, as though one were peeling a banana or rolling up a sleeve (Fig 3). The end point is circumferentially visible at the end of the everted artery. Loose pieces of media and intima are picked or shaved off the wall.

After endarterectomy of the CCA and ECA is completed, the unrolled artery is held up to the arteriotomy in the CCA. The cephalad ends of both arteriotomies should be opposed. If the ICA is redundant, the proximal end may be amputated; otherwise, the common carotid arteriotomy is extended proximally so that the end of this arteriotomy can oppose the proximal end of the endarterectomized ICA. The 2 arteriotomies are typically 15 to 30 mm long at this time. Endarterectomy of the CCA and ECA is done in the same fashion as conventional endarterectomy. A fine monofilament nonabsorbable suture (6-0 is usually ideal) is used to reattach the ICA to the distal

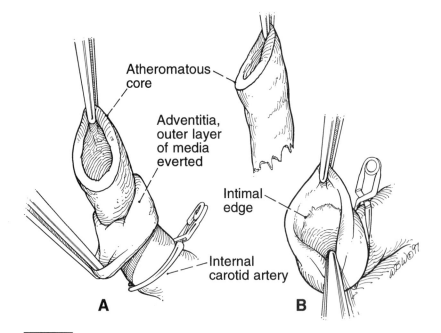

FIGURE 3.

A, Removal of plaque and **B**, visualization of end point. (Copyright 1997, William B. Westwood.)

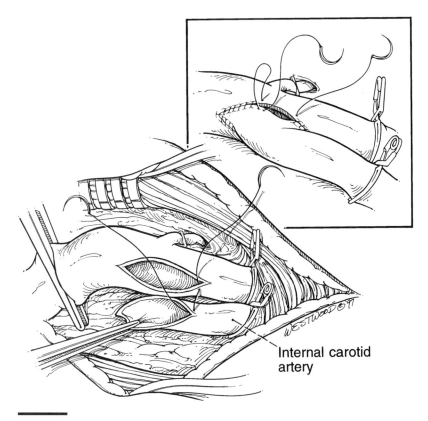

Internal carotid
artery

FIGURE 4.

Reanastomosis of internal to common carotid artery. (Copyright 1997, William B. Westwood.)

CCA. The suture is usually started at the most cephalad ends of both arteriotomies, and the 2 ends are brought around as desired (Fig 4).

A major advantage of eversion endarterectomy is that the arteriotomies are large and the lumens are used to "patch" each other. By removing one of the major technical issues of CEA, eversion endarterectomy obviates the need for tedious primary closure of the distal ICA. The clamps may be flashed and the lumen irrigated before the suture line is completed. After completion, flow is instituted into the ECA before unclamping the ICA. With all arteries unclamped, the flow is assessed by Doppler and the patient observed for neurologic changes. Our average carotid cross-clamp time is 14.7 ± 4.7 minutes (range, 9-21 minutes) on each side. The neck incisions are closed with suction drains after the completion of the coronary revascularization.

INTRAOPERATIVE CAROTID SHUNTS

At our institution, CEA is routinely performed with the patients awake, and we have adopted the principle of selective shunting in those who do not tolerate brief carotid clamping. However, all the bilateral CEA/CABG procedures are done with the patients under general anesthesia. Initially, we measured stump pressures and shunted patients if the pressure was less than 40 mm Hg. We have purposefully not used a shunt in the last 59 bilateral CEA/CABG patients, without any changed outcome. Probably the most frequent objection to eversion endarterectomy is that shunting is difficult or impossible. This has not been our experience. That said, certain shunts do work better than others with eversion. Shunts fixed at either end with either an internal balloon (Pruitt-Inahara type) or with external clamping (Javid type) are most suitable for eversion techniques. Once in place, they may actually make eversion of the distal ICA easier. Unfortunately, straight shunts are not usable because traction on the arteries results in dislodgment.

Shunt insertion may be accomplished in the following fashion. After the ICA is divided from the CCA and mobilized, the arteriotomy is extended cephalad a variable distance. In some cases, this extension goes through the end point, and normal lumen is visible. A shunt can be inserted at this time. Alternatively, if the end point of the plaque is not encompassed by the arteriotomy, the plaque is everted and removed to expose the normal lumen. Shunt insertion now may be performed. Although the second method may seem time-consuming, shunt insertion may usually be accomplished in less than a minute after initial clamping of the arteries. Proximal insertion of a shunt is facilitated by the usual caudal extension of the common carotid arteriotomy.

After flow is established in the shunt, the ICA is everted over the shunt. If the clamp is placed cephalad enough, the shunt acts as a mandrel over which the artery is everted (Fig 5). Endarterectomy of the CCA is completed in standard fashion with the shunt in place by the methods previously described. Reanastomosis is accomplished by completing as much of the suture line as possible while leaving the shunt protruding from the anterior surface. The shunt is then removed, the arteries are reclamped, and the suture line is completed in the standard fashion.

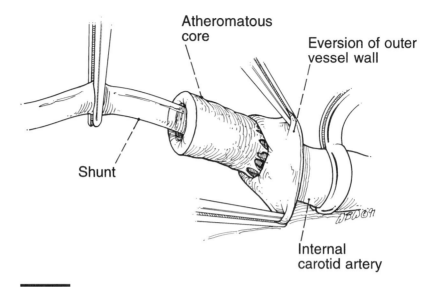

FIGURE 5.

Eversion of adventitia over intraluminal shunt. (Copyright 1997, William B. Westwood.)

POSTOPERATIVE CARE

During the immediate postoperative period, both vascular and cardiothoracic surgical teams monitor the patients. Cardiac care is administered by the cardiothoracic surgeon in conjunction with a cardiologist. In-hospital morbidity and mortality for each patient is documented. A neurology consult is obtained in all patients with any abnormal findings. A major neurologic event is defined as the recognition of a new motor or sensory neurologic deficit, as well as the correlation of symptoms with radiologic signs on computed tomographic or magnetic resonance imaging of the head. The patient is extubated and evaluated for any vocal cord paralysis as well as for respiratory compromise. On postoperative day 1, the cervical drains are removed. Patients are followed up with serial duplex ultrasound examinations at 6-month intervals.

SHORT- AND LONG-TERM RESULTS AND COMPLICATIONS

Between January 1994 and February 2002, we performed 67 bilateral CEA/CABG procedures. All patients had New York Heart Class 4 angina with bilateral carotid artery stenosis of 80% or more who were scheduled to undergo CABG. There were 35 men and 32 women (mean age, 69 years, range, 48-88 years).

Perioperative risk factors were diabetes (n = 17, 25%) and a history of smoking (n = 30, 45%). Two patients (2%) had a prior history of stroke, 13 (10%) had transient ischemic attacks, and 6 (5%) had amaurosis fugax. No patient was symptomatic from both carotid arteries. Twenty-one patients (31%) had a symptomatic lesion.

The average cross-clamp time for each carotid artery was 14.7 ± 4.7 minutes (range, 9-21 minutes), and the total perfusion time was 123 ± 29 minutes (range, 77-183 minutes). The mean number of coronary bypass grafts was 4 ± 1 per patient. The average length of stay in the cardiopulmonary intensive care unit was 4 ± 14 days (median, 1 day; range, 1-100 days), and the total hospital stay was 6 to 100 days. No permanent or transient neurologic events were observed in the early postoperative period. Nonfatal postoperative complications occurred in 10% (7/67) of patients. No patient had respiratory failure secondary to vocal cord paralysis, consistent with findings we previously reported.[23]

Perioperative mortality occurred in 3 of 67 patients (4.5%). Two of these 3 patients had mitral valve insufficiency associated with a severely depressed left ventricular fraction (<30%). One of them developed methicillin-resistant *Staphylococcus aureus* endocarditis of the native mitral valve 2 months after operation and eventually died of multiorgan system failure. Respiratory failure, gastrointestinal bleeding, and sepsis from methicillin-resistant *S aureus* pneumonia complicated this patient's perioperative course. Another patient who had a combined CABG/CEA along with a posterior mitral annuloplasty had low cardiac output syndrome postoperatively, requiring prolonged use of an intra-aortic balloon pump. Complications of respiratory failure, renal failure, and sepsis from infectious colitis eventually resulted in this patient's death. One patient died as a result of a postoperative stroke.

SUMMARY

Patients who have significant coronary artery disease associated with symptomatic or asymptomatic bilateral carotid artery occlusive disease may be considered for simultaneous bilateral CEA and coronary revascularization. This combined operation can be performed with an acceptable overall mortality and morbidity rate. No patient in this series or in a prior series of 256 patients undergoing staged bilateral CEA without CABG had respiratory failure from vocal cord paralysis.[23] Nonetheless, severe left ventricular dysfunction or severe mitral valve disease is not the exclusion criterion for performing concomitant bilateral CEA/CABG. The mortality rate in our series of 67 bilateral CEA/CABG operations was 4.5%. One of the 3 deaths was technical (thrombosis of the ICA), resulting in a postoperative stroke. Although the mortality rate in our series is higher than that for standard open-heart procedures, it is comparable to that reported in the literature for simultaneous unilateral CEA and coronary revascularization.[21] Of note, patients with depressed left ventricular function and concomitant valvular pathology contributed to a higher mortality rate in patients undergoing bilateral CEA/CABG. On the other hand, the presence of bilateral symptomatic or asymptomatic carotid artery disease was not found to be a significant risk factor for increased neurologic events or mortality in our patient population.

REFERENCES

1. Dylewski, M, Canver CC, Chanda J, et al: Coronary artery bypass combined with bilateral carotid endarterectomy. *Ann Thorac Surg* 71:777-782, 2001.
2. Mackey WC, Khabbaz K, Bojar R, et al: Simultaneous carotid endarterectomy and coronary bypass: Perioperative risk and long-term survival. *J Vasc Surg* 24:58-64, 1996.
3. Faggioli GL, Curl GR, Ricotta JJ, et al: The role of carotid screening before coronary artery bypass. *J Vasc Surg* 12:724-731, 1990.
4. Rizzo RJ, Whittemore AD, Couper GS, et al: Combined carotid and coronary revascularization: The preferred approach to the severe vasculopath. *Ann Thorac Surg* 54:1099-1109, 1992.
5. Chang BB, Darling RC III, Shah DM, et al: Carotid endarterectomy can be safely performed with acceptable mortality and morbidity in patients requiring coronary artery bypass grafts. *Am J Surg* 168:94-96, 1994.
6. Brener BJ, Brief DK, Alpert J, et al: The risk of stroke in patients with asymptomatic carotid stenosis undergoing cardiac surgery: A follow up study. *J Vasc Surg* 5:269-277, 1987.
7. Abrishamchian AR, Darling RC III, Roddy SP, et al: Combined coronary artery bypass with carotid endarterectomy. Do women have worse outcomes? *J Vasc Surg*, in press.
8. Furlan AJ, Cracium AR: Risk of stroke during coronary artery bypass graft surgery in patients with internal carotid artery disease documented by angiography. *Stroke* 16:797-799, 1985.
9. Pome G, Passini L, Colucci V, et al: Combined surgical approach to coexistent carotid and coronary artery disease. *J Cardiovasc Surg* 32:787-793, 1992.
10. Kouchoukos NT, Daily BB, Wareing TH, et al: Hypothermic circulatory arrest for cerebral protection during combined carotid and cardiac surgery in patients with bilateral carotid artery disease. *Ann Surg* 6:699-706, 1994.

11. Nunn DD. Carotid endarterectomy: An analysis of 204 operative cases. *Ann Surg* 182:733-740, 1975.

12. Hertzer NR, Loop FD, Beven EG, et al: Surgical staging for simultaneous coronary and carotid disease: A study including prospective randomization. *J Vasc Surg* 9:455-463, 1989.

13. Breslau PJ, Fell G, Ivey TD, et al: Carotid arterial disease in patients undergoing coronary artery bypass operations. *J Thorac Cardiovasc Surg* 82:765-767, 1981.

14. Senseing DM: Bilateral carotid endarterectomy at one operation. *J Maine Med Assoc* 65:304-305, 1974.

15. Clauss RH, Bole PV, Paredes M, et al: Simultaneous bilateral carotid endarterectomies. *Arch Surg* 111:1304-1306, 1976.

16. De Geest R, Bast TJ, Eikelboom BC, et al: One stage operation of bilateral carotid lesions. *Acta Chir Belg* 78:95-102, 1979.

17. Clauss RH, Babu SC, Patel KR, et al: Simultaneous carotid endarterectomy operations. *J Cardiovasc Surg* 26:297-299, 1985.

18. Dimakos PB, Kotsis T, Tsiligiris B, et al: Comparative results of staged and simultaneous bilateral carotid endarterectomy: A clinical study and surgical treatment. *Cardiovasc Surg* 8:10-17, 2000.

19. Mulinari LA, Tyszka AL, Silva AZ, et al: Bilateral carotid endarterectomy combined with myocardial revascularization during the same surgical act. *Arq Bras Cardiol* 74:353-354, 2000.

20. Al-Mubarak N, Roubin GS, Vitek JJ, et al: Simultaneous bilateral carotid stenting for restenosis after endarterectomy. *Cathet Cardiovasc Diagn* 45:11-15, 1988.

21. Darling RC III, Dylewski MR, Chang BB, et al: Combined carotid endarterectomy and coronary artery bypass grafting does not increase the risk of perioperative strokes. *Cardiovasc Surg* 6:4484-4452, 1998.

22. Taylor DC, Strandness DE: Carotid artery duplex scanning. *J Clin Ultrasound* 15:635-644, 1987.

23. Ozsvath KJ, Darling RC III, Kreienberg PB, et al: Is clinical exam an adequate predictor of respiratory dysfunction after bilateral carotid endarterectomy. *Vasc Surg* 33:447-450, 1999.

CHAPTER 4

Surgical Management of Carotid Body Tumors

Giuseppe R. Nigri, MD, PhD
Clinical Fellow in Surgery, Department of Surgery, Massachusetts General Hospital, Harvard Medical School, Boston, Mass

Glenn M. LaMuraglia, MD
Associate Professor of Surgery, Division of Vascular Surgery, Massachusetts General Hospital, Harvard Medical School, Boston, Mass

Carotid body tumors (CBTs), also known as chemodectomas or cervical paragangliomas, arise from neural crest cells at the carotid bifurcation. These slow-growing tumors are highly vascular, densely adherent to the carotid bifurcation, and can encompass the cranial nerves. The surgical treatment of CBTs, even if improved during the last century, is still considered challenging. The highly vascular nature of the tumors, their adherence to the vessel wall, and their proximity to the cranial nerves can result in a high morbidity related mainly to cranial nerve damage.[1] For these reasons, it is mandatory to carefully select these patients for surgical resection. In specific circumstances, decreasing the vascularity of the tumor before surgery is very helpful. In addition, meticulous surgical technique is of paramount importance to minimize the neurologic complications.

EPIDEMIOLOGY

CBTs are rare, and only 1400 cases of these tumors have been reported in the literature.[2,3] These tumors have the same frequency in males and females and are usually diagnosed in the fourth and fifth decade of life. Their presentation can be sporadic (80%) or familial (20%).[4] In the more common sporadic form of the disease, tumors are present bilaterally in 5% of cases.[5] In the familial form, they are transmitted as an autosomal dominant with complete penetrance. In these instances, they can be bilateral (32%-00%), often associated with other paragangliomas, such as pheochromocytomas.[3] These tumors can also be part of multiple endocrine neoplasia (MEN I and II). For these reasons, patients with CBTs should have a complete preoperative evaluation to verify the presence of associated tumors. They should also be counseled for family member screening because of the high relative incidence in family members. There is a controversial relationship between CBTs and exposure to chronic hypoxia.[5] This has been inferred because of the higher incidence of CBTs in persons living at high altitudes (such as the Andes) or in those with chronic obstructive pulmonary disease.

PATHOLOGY AND BIOLOGIC BEHAVIOR

CBTs consist of nests of neuroectodermal cells (zellballen) that contain neuroendocrine granules of serotonin, epinephrine, and norepinephrine. However, only rarely (5%) are CBTs functioning tumors, causing hypertension.[5] Grossly, they are usually well-circumscribed, highly vascularized, reddish brown, rubbery lesions. However, they do not have a true capsule and can adhere tenaciously to the adventitia of the carotid artery. Malignancy has been reported in about 10% of CBTs (range, 2%-50%), but there are no large series of malignant CBTs, and not many have been recently reported. Malignancy cannot be predicted based on cell morphology or mitotic activity, and therefore the mass should always be completed excised when possible to avoid local and distal recurrence. The hallmark for the diagnosis of malignancy is lymph node involvement or distant metastases (kidney, thyroid, pancreas, cerebellum, lungs, bone, etc). Metastases can develop many years after original resection but are rare. Therefore, continued vigilance of these patients should be undertaken.

Even though CBTs are slow-growing tumors, they can enlarge and splay the carotid arteries and distort the anatomy of the carotid bifurcation. The size of these tumors influences the surgical outcome. In fact, the larger the tumor, the more frequent are the complications (cranial nerve injury, bleeding) because of the increase in the complexity of surgical manipulation. The Shamblin classification,[6] which relates the complexity of surgical dissection to the size of tumors and involvement of adjacent structures, even if rarely used in a clinical setting, still maintains a historical importance. Shamblin type I includes small tumors that are easily resected from the carotid bifurcation (Fig 1, A). The type II tumors are more adherent to the arteries and can partially surround them (Fig 1, B). Shamblin type III includes all tumors that encase the carotid arteries and possibly the

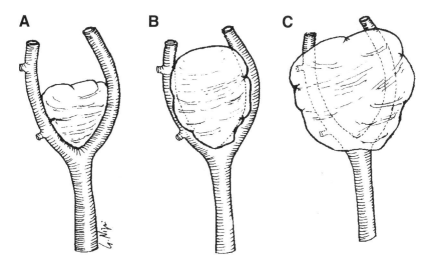

FIGURE 1.
The Shamblin classification. **A,** Shamblin type I includes small tumors that are easily resected from the carotid bifurcation. **B,** Type II tumors are more adherent to the arteries and can partially surround them. **C,** Type III tumors encase the carotid arteries and possibly the nerves and often require surgical resection and subsequent vessel reconstruction.

nerves, and often require surgical resection and subsequent vessel reconstruction (Fig 1, C).

CLINICAL PRESENTATION AND DIAGNOSIS

The tumor usually appears as an asymptomatic mass at the mandibular angle. Sometimes the patient notes a lump in the lateral neck that has been slowly growing over several years. The mass is usually mobile laterally but fixed on the vertical plane, because of the adherence to the carotid artery (Fontaine's sign).[7] It can appear pulsatile but not expansive, and sometimes a systolic bruit can be heard over the bifurcation. In contrast, carotid aneurysms appear both pulsatile and expansive, although this can be difficult to determine on physical examination. Since the mass can involve the vagus and the glossopharyngeal nerves as well as the sympathetic chain, symptoms related to their dysfunction can sometimes be noticed. The patient may complain about neck pain, local tenderness, dysphagia, and voice changes. Manipulation of the tumor can result in a decrease of heart rate and dizziness. In those patients in whom the tumor secretes catecholamines (5%), palpitations, tachycardia, arrhythmias,

TABLE 1.
Differential Diagnosis

Benign nodal inflammation or hypertrophy

Brachial cleft cyst
Carotid aneurysm
Glomus jugulare tumor
Low parotid tumor
Lymphoma
Metastatic cancer to a cervical node
Submandibular salivary gland tumor
Thyroid lesion

dizziness, headache, flushing, and diaphoresis have been reported. In these cases, further evaluation and careful planning of anesthesia are mandatory.

An accurate history and physical examination can help to rule out other causes of cervical masses (Table 1). Preoperative evaluation of large tumors should include indirect laryngoscopy and careful documentation of vocal cord function, and neurologic examination of the other cranial nerves. Catecholamine levels should be measured in patients with suspected functionally active CBTs and in those with bilateral tumors. In addition, iodine 131 (^{131}I)-meta-iodobenzylguanidine scan can determine the functional state of the tumor and the presence of associated paragangliomas[4]; however, this modality is rarely used clinically.

IMAGING

Color-flow ultrasonography is a noninvasive, cost-effective imaging technique that can make the initial diagnosis of CBT. The typical sonographic features include a poorly echogenic mass, splaying the carotid bifurcation, in which pulsed Doppler analysis can demonstrate arterial waveforms with a turbulent low-resistance flow pattern.[4] This imaging modality may exclude a CBT or other vascular entity that may be mistaken for a malignant head and neck tumor. Therefore, this could avoid an ill-advised biopsy procedure, which could result in significant hemorrhage. In addition, color-flow ultrasonography is highly effective in screening of both sporadic and familial cases. It is useful in early detection, diagnostic confirmation, and demonstration of any associated carotid stenotic lesion, and can be used for follow-up of nonoperatively managed or postoperative resection of CBT. If the patient findings are not characteristic of CBT, or Doppler color-flow ultrasonography does not confirm the diagnosis, patients should be referred for a comprehensive ear-nose-throat evaluation, since other causes of cervical masses can be confused with CBTs (Table 1).

Computed tomography (CT) with and without contrast can be useful in assessing size and cranial extension of the tumor,[7] and it has been largely used for Shamblin classification of CBTs. However, CT scan alone cannot distinguish between CBT and carotid aneurysm (Fig 2), which can be done by color-flow ultrasonography or arteriography.

Magnetic resonance imaging (MRI) does give comparable results to CT scan and is more expensive. Magnetic resonance angiography (MRA) has been recently advocated, since the imaging of both carotid and vertebral arteries can be obtained. With the latest software technology for 3-dimensional reconstruction, CT and MRI of these highly vascularized tumors allow the detection of multicentric and bilateral tumors or other associated paragangliomas of the neck.

Indium 111 (^{111}In)-pentetreotide scintigraphy is another noninvasive imaging modality for locating neuroendocrine tumors. It is a nuclear medicine scan that when performed of the whole body can detect tumor location, multicentricity, residual tumor after excision, recurrence, and metastases. The images are based on the tumor's properties of containing somatostatin receptors, and that ^{111}In-pentetreotide mimics the action of somatostatin.[8] This has been considered to be a useful method to screen for the location of multicentric paragangliomas.

Traditionally, bilateral angiography has been considered the "gold standard" for the diagnosis of CBT. Color-flow ultrasonography, CT, MRI, and MRA have decreased the necessity for this invasive technique for small tumors. However, angiography still maintains a central role in evaluating large and highly vascularized masses. It can also demonstrate the presence of multicentric disease, and is especially useful to delineate concurrent atherosclerosis and feeding vessels of the CBT. In addition, this diagnostic tool can be transformed into an interventional technique in the instances that embolization of the tumor blood supply would be necessary.

PREOPERATIVE EMBOLIZATION

The tumor, which is highly vascularized, usually receives its blood supply from the external carotid artery branches, mainly through the ascending pharyngeal artery. However, when the tumor grows, its vascular supply can develop from the internal carotid artery, vertebral artery, and thyrocervical trunk. The high vascularity (Fig 3, A and B) and the intimate relationship with the carotid artery and cra-

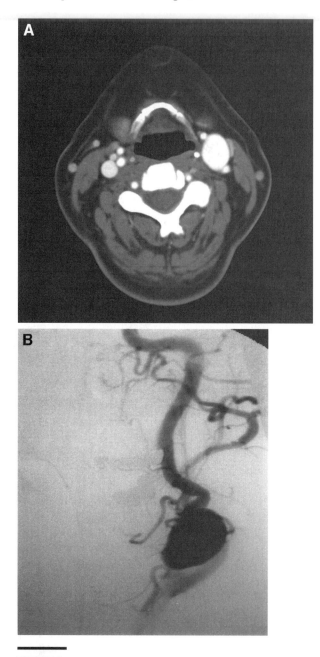

FIGURE 2.

Carotid aneurysm. **A,** CT alone cannot distinguish between a carotid aneurysm or a CBT. **B,** Arteriography is necessary to determine the nature of the lesion.

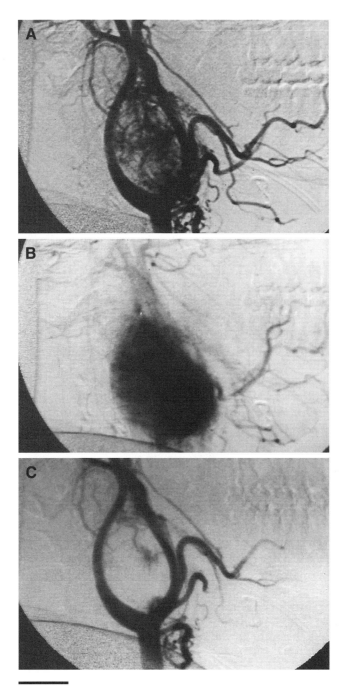

FIGURE 3.
A, Arteriography of the carotid vessels and CBT. **B,** Blushing of the tumor is visible after contrast injection. **C,** The tumor blushing disappears after embolization.

nial nerves render the exclsion of this tumor a true surgical challenge. Because it is not possible to reduce the vascularity of the CBT intraoperatively, large tumors predicate the necessity of preoperative embolization. Embolization should be considered to reduce vascularity (Fig 3, C), consequently decreasing blood loss and facilitating surgery, which can translate into lower morbidity. The embolization is recommended in tumors larger than 3 cm, whereas it may not be worth the risk in smaller tumors.[9] CBT embolization can run the risk of stroke and should be performed only by highly qualified personnel. Embolization is performed by slow injection of polyvinyl alcohol beads immersed in contrast into the vasculature of the tumor. Only the vessels that can be directly catheterized are embolized, to avoid reflux of particles into the cerebral, vertebral, or ophthalmic circulation.[10] Once the blood flow to the feeder vessels is significantly reduced, a gelatin sponge or a coil is deployed at the vessel origin to induce thrombosis. Particular attention has to be given to the "dangerous anastomoses," which are collateral branches from the feeding vessels that anastomose to the vertebral or internal carotid artery[9] and provide direct access to the cerebral circulation. Embolization of these vessels is contraindicated to avoid embolization of the brain. In addition, the initial injection of opacified lidocaine into the vessels while neurologic examination is performed can be useful to avoid embolization of vessels perfusing cranial nerves. To avoid edema and inflammation of the area, it is suggested to perform surgery within 48 hours.

SURGICAL MANAGEMENT

The patient lies supine, with the neck extended facing the contralateral side of the CBT. One leg should be prepared for surgery because, if surgical resection of the carotid vessels is needed, the saphenous vein can be used during reconstruction. General anesthesia is used, preferentially with nasotracheal intubation, since this provides easier jaw manipulation, especially if mandibular subluxation is considered to improve exposure for very large tumors. Electroencephalography, even if not mandatory, can be helpful in assessing the cerebral circulation should carotid clamping and reconstruction be necessary. Carotid shunting is only undertaken if there are positive elecroencephalographic changes or if no cerebral monitoring is available.

The surgical approach is through an oblique neck incision anterior to the sternocleidomastoid muscle. A "T" or "Y" incision can be used in the case of large tumors that extend cranially, toward the base of the skull. In these cases, subluxation of the temporomandibular joint can be used to better expose the cephalad portion of the tumor.[11] Mobilization of the parotid gland and retraction of the digastric and stylohyoid muscles are easiest, but their division may be necessary to facilitate high exposure of the CBT.[2] Meticulous dissection and use of bipolar electrocautery are very helpful to avoid damaging surrounding structures, such as cranial nerves. The initial part of the dissection should be the identification of the vagus and hypoglossal nerves, so they can be protected during the operation. The proximal and distal control of the carotid vessels should be performed, even if these maneuvers are often very difficult when large tumors are present.[12] Dissection of the CBT off the carotid artery should be carried out in the periadventitial space, starting at the superior anterior margin of the tumor, working toward the bifurcation, and extending caudally onto the posterior aspects of the internal and external carotid arteries. This kind of dissection can be performed in Shamblin stage I and II tumors. Stage III tumors often require resection of the involved portion and vessel resulting in carotid reconstruction, preferentially with the saphenous vein when available.[2] In very difficult cases, early division of the external carotid artery facilitates dissection, especially at the bifurcation, and reconstruction of the external carotid artery usually is not necessary. CBT resection does not require lymph node dissection. However, the sampling of regional lymph nodes for metastases has been proposed.[3] A 2-team approach, including vascular and head and neck surgeons, has been advocated, especially in larger tumors.

COMPLICATIONS

Historically, CBT surgery has resulted in high rates of morbidity (40%) and mortality (29%) related to the bleeding and cranial nerve involvement.[4] This has significantly improved, and most recent series have shown low mortality rates (0.6%-2%) and a significant decrease in morbidity rates (10%-20%).[4] These complications need to be considered when deciding whether to resect a CBT, in addition to considering the patient's comorbid risk factors, tumor size, and tumor involvement of adjacent structures, and the slow-growing nature of the tumor.

Major blood loss has been reported during surgical resection of CBTs,[13] sometimes requiring a mean of 2.1 units of blood replacement or more in nonanemic patients.[14,15] However, other series showed that blood transfusion was only rarely needed, in particular after preoperative embolization of CBTs.[9]

Cranial nerve damage still remains the most frequent complication, even today. The nerves at risk include cranial nerves VII, IX, X, and XII, and the sympathetic trunk (Horner syndrome).[1] Cranial nerves X and XII are the most common cranial nerves subject to injury during large tumor dissection. The isolated loss of cranial nerve X affects the vocal cords, swallowing, and protection of the airway, depending on the level of injury. When combined with the loss of other cranial nerves, the function of the upper aerodigestive tract can be significantly impaired.[16] The stroke rate during CBT surgery is low and has been reported to be about 1.9%,[4] but these strokes are generally minor.

The surgeon's decision regarding whether to resect the CBT is based on the consideration of these possible complications and the health status of the individual patient. However, in experienced hands, most patients are operative candidates. In rare instances, palliative treatment should be considered. In this case, radiotherapy has been suggested by some, but this therapy is highly controversial. Although some studies describe CBTs as radioresistant,[17,18] with radiotherapy offering no benefit to the patient, others studies have shown radiotherapy to offer modest benefit.[3,7] Patients not undergoing surgical therapy should be followed up every 6 months for tumor growth and evidence of compression symptoms of adjacent structures. Patients who have undergone carotid artery reconstruction should be monitored every 6 months for a 2-year period to evaluate the development of a stenotic lesion in the bypass. In addition, follow-up of those patients who undergo surgery has to be considered because of the possibility of metachronous lesions. For this reason these patients and their relatives should be monitored for the appearance of new lesions.

REFERENCES

1. Plukker JT, Brongers EP, Vermey A, et al: Outcome of surgical treatment for carotid body paraganglioma. *Br J Surg* 88:1382-1386, 2001.
2. Westerband A, Hunter GC, Cintora I, et al: Current trends in the detection and management of carotid body tumors. *J Vasc Surg* 28:84-92, 1998; discussion pp 92-93.
3. Dias Da Silva A, O'Donnell S, Gillespie D, et al: Malignant carotid body tumor: A case report. *J Vasc Surg* 32:821-823, 2000.
4. Muhm M, Polterauer P, Gstottner W, et al: Diagnostic and therapeutic approaches to carotid body tumors. Review of 24 patients. *Arch Surg* 132:279-284, 1997.
5. Hallett JW Jr, Nora JD, Hollier LH, et al: Trends in neurovascular complications of surgical management for carotid body and cervical paragangliomas: A fifty-year experience with 153 tumors. *J Vasc Surg* 7:284-291, 1988.

6. Shamblin WR, ReMine WH, Sheps SG, et al: Carotid body tumor (chemodectoma). Clinicopathologic analysis of ninety cases. *Am J Surg* 122:732-739, 1971.
7. Dickinson PR, Griffin SM, Guy AJ, et al: Carotid body tumour: 30 years experience. *Br J Surg* 73:14-16, 1986.
8. Hammond SL, Greco DL, Lambert AT, et al: Indium In-111 pentetreotide scintigraphy: Application to carotid body tumors. *J Vasc Surg* 25:905-908, 1997.
9. LaMuraglia GM, Fabian RL, Brewster DC, et al: The current surgical management of carotid body paragangliomas. *J Vasc Surg* 15:1038-1044, 1992; discussion pp 1044-1045.
10. Brismar J, Cronqvist S: Therapeutic embolization in the external carotid artery region. *Acta Radiol Diagn* 19:715-731, 1978.
11. Dossa C, Shepard AD, Wolford DG, et al: Distal internal carotid exposure: A simplified technique for temporary mandibular subluxation. *J Vasc Surg* 12:319-325, 1990.
12. Meyer FB, Sundt TM Jr, Pearson BW: Carotid body tumors: A subject review and suggested surgical approach. *J Neurosurg* 64:377-385, 1986.
13. Kafie FE, Freischlag JA: Carotid body tumors: The role of preoperative embolization. *Ann Vasc Surg* 15:237-242, 2001.
14. Rosen IB, Palmer JA, Goldberg M, et al: Vascular problems associated with carotid body tumors. *Am J Surg* 142:459-463, 1981.
15. Dent TL, Thompson NW, Fry WJ: Carotid body tumors. *Surgery* 80:365-372, 1976.
16. Sniezek JC, Sabri AN, Netterville JL: Paraganglioma surgery: Complications and treatment. *Otolaryngol Clin North Am* 34:993-1006, 2001.
17. Valdagni R, Amichetti M: Radiation therapy of carotid body tumors. *Am J Clin Oncol* 13:45-48, 1990.
18. Martin CE, Rosenfeld L, McSwain B: Carotid body tumors: A 16-year follow-up of seven malignant cases. *South Med J* 66:1236-1243, 1973.

Part II

Aortic Disease

CHAPTER 5

Treatment of Abdominal Aortic Aneurysms With the Ancure Endograft System

Victor M. Bernhard, MD

Lecturer in Vascular Surgery, University of Chicago, Pritzker School of Medicine, Chicago, Ill

The application of endograft exclusion for the definitive treatment of abdominal aortic aneurysm (AAA) has increased dramatically since 2 devices achieved Food and Drug Administration (FDA) approval for market in September 1999. As expected with any new approach to management, there has been an increasingly vigorous debate regarding the use of this technique as an alternative to standard open surgical repair (SOR). The recommendation for the endovascular approach rather than conventional surgery depends on the anatomic constraints imposed by the design of the specific endograft and its delivery system, the early outcomes reported for the insertion procedure, and the long-term prevention of aneurysm rupture without adverse side effects when compared with SOR.

The Ancure Endograft System, the most recent version of the device produced by the Endovascular Solutions Division of the Guidant Corporation, is one of the devices currently approved for commercial use in the United States. This chapter presents the results of the clinical application of this device to date and compares these outcomes with a control group of patients who were treated concurrently by SOR of their aneurysms.

HISTORY OF THE ANCURE DEVICE

Endovascular Technologies designed and tested the second generation of the tube and bifurcation endografts in 1995. Thereafter, the FDA granted Investigative Device Exemptions for phase 2 and 3 clinical trials of these devices, and the investigations were completed in 1999. In September 1999, Guidant Corp, the successor to Endovascular Technologies, received approval to market these endograft systems with the provision that the clinical trial patients would be followed up for 5 years under a standardized surveillance protocol. The currently available devices, designated as Ancure, have the same tube and bifurcation implant designs as those used in the phase 2 and 3 clinical trials; however, the delivery catheter has been slightly modified to simplify graft delivery.

More than 10,000 patients have been treated with Ancure endografts since the pre-market approval (PMA) was received. A temporary recall of all devices was initiated by the company in March 2001 because of inadequacies in reporting the application of newly developed techniques to facilitate endograft delivery, undocumented modifications in the instructions for use, and a concern for the reliability of device packaging. From March 19 to April 13, 2001, the company, with FDA approval, carried out a short-term study of the currently marketed endografts to evaluate the immediate results of implant deployment with these modified techniques. There were no adverse outcomes, and after resolution of the aforementioned issues, the Ancure devices were reapproved for market in August 2001.

The phase 2 trial for the aorto-monoiliac (A-I) variant of the Ancure device was completed in 2001, and the results of this investigation have been submitted to the FDA.

DEVICE DESCRIPTION

The Ancure device is available in tube, bifurcation, and A-I configurations (Fig 1, A-C). The endograft itself is composed of a woven polyester fabric that is crimped in the iliac limb segments of the bifurcation and monoiliac grafts. The attachment systems are fashioned from the metal alloy Elgiloy, and are sutured to the proximal and distal ends of the endograft. The aortic attachment system consists of 2 components: a self-expanding stent with a "Z" configuration, and a series of paired hooks spaced equidistantly around the circumference (Fig 1, D). A modified version of this system is used to attach the iliac limbs. The stent provides the lateral expansion force to produce a circumferential seal of the graft material against the arterial wall and hook penetration to prevent graft migration from the attachment sites. All configurations of the endograft have a unibody construction without additional modules and with no supporting stents or struts between the proximal and distal attachment systems. The body of the tube graft and the aortic portions of the bifurcation and monoiliac variants are available in 20- to 26-mm di-

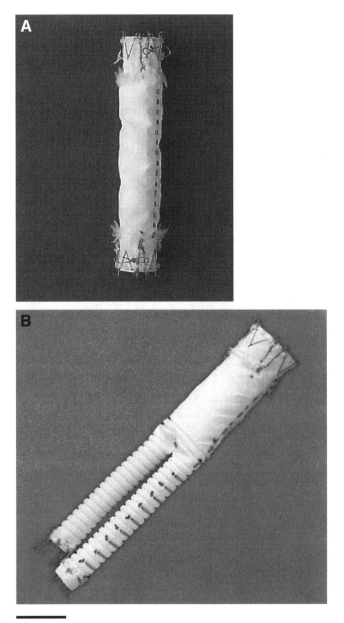

FIGURE 1.

The 3 configurations of the Ancure endograft system: **(A)** tube, **(B)** bifurca-

(continued)

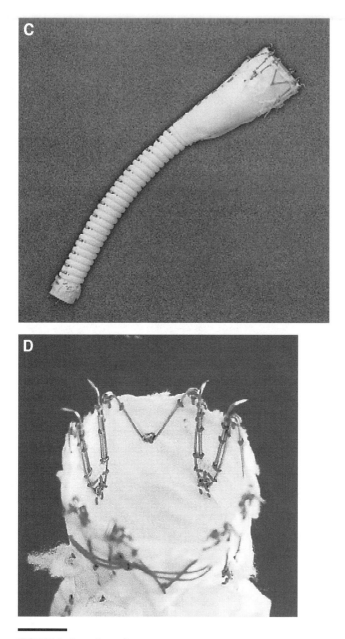

FIGURE 1. (continued)
tion, **(C)** aorto-monoiliac, and **(D)** the hook-bearing aortic attachment
system.

ameters. The iliac limb segments of the bifurcation and monoiliac designs vary in diameter from 10 to 13 mm.

The A-I system is reserved for those patients in whom the anatomy of one iliac artery prohibits effective positioning of a limb of the bifurcation graft. After insertion of the aorto-uni-iliac endograft, the contralateral common iliac artery, if it is not already obstructed by atherosclerosis, must be closed with coils or other occluding device to prevent back flow into the aneurysm.[1] Thereafter, circulation to the contralateral extremity is restored with a femorofemoral bypass.

The delivery system consists of a coaxial catheter, 23.5F in diameter, with the endograft compressed within its proximal end. The device is introduced through a common femoral arteriotomy over a stiff guidewire for delivery of the implant at the site of the AAA. Balloon expansion is used to assist penetration of the attachment hooks into the walls of the aortic neck and iliac arteries to ensure an effective seal and endograft fixation. For delivery of the bifurcation endograft, an additional pull-wire, attached to the contralateral graft limb, is passed through the ipsilateral femoral artery along with the main delivery catheter. It is advanced to the aortic bifurcation where it is captured by a snare and withdrawn from the contralateral femoral artery. This wire is used to position the contralateral graft limb in the iliac artery and deploy its attachment system.

CLINICAL TRIALS

The data relating to the Ancure endograft were derived from clinical trials approved and monitored by the FDA.[2,3] Short-term outcomes were obtained from all patients entered into phase 2 and 3 investigations between November 1995 and September 1999. These included 197 patients who were enrolled to be treated with tube, 573 patients to be treated with bifurcation, and 121 patients to receive A-I grafts. A control group for all 3 versions of the Ancure device consisted of 111 patients who were treated concurrently with standard open aneurysm repair.

The postmarket study, performed in March and April 2001, enrolled 361 patients for treatment with bifurcation endografts to evaluate the immediate outcomes of modifications in deployment methodology.[4] These patients were not entered into a long-term evaluation protocol.

Long-term follow-up evaluation for 5 years was mandated by the FDA as a requirement for market approval for all patients in phase 2 and a portion of those in phase 3 of the tube and bifurcation trials. The long-term data beyond 1 year for the A-I endograft system are currently under review by the FDA and are unavailable for publication at this time.

EARLY RESULTS

The early results (<30 days) from the phase 2 and 3 trails for all 3 configurations of the current version of the Ancure device and for the post-PMA bifurcation study are summarized in Table 1. The operative mortality rate was low for all device types and was similar to that of the control group. Deployment success, based on intent to treat, was achieved in more than 91% of patients in the clinical trials and increased to 95% in the more recent postmarket bifurcation study. The better success rate noted in this latter group of bifurcation grafts that was evaluated 18 months after market release probably represents improved case selection and the application of refinements in the techniques of endograft deployment. For all graft configurations, failure to achieve endograft implantation was most commonly caused by an inability to gain access through the iliac arteries.

Major operative complications were reduced significantly for patients treated with tube and bifurcation endografts when com-

TABLE 1.

Perioperative Results (Implant to 30 Days) for the Ancure Tube, Bifurcation, and A-I Endografts Under FDA Clinical Trials and a Later Postmarket Approval Bifurcation Endograft Study *(Right Column)*

	Tube	Bifurcation	A-I	Control	P*	Bifurcation Postmarket
N (No. attempted)	197	573	121	111	—	361
Perioperative Mortality (%)	0	1.7	4.2	2.7	NS	1.7
Successful implant (%)	92.4	91.2	91	NA	—	95
Major complications (%)	19.8*	28.7*	35.6	44.1	<.001	—
Median operative blood loss (mL)	200*	300*	400*	800	<.001	—
ICU care (%)	35.5*	39.1*	38.6*	96.3	.005	—
Operative time (min)	156	159	258*	174	.001	—
Median postoperative stay (d) (median)	2*	3*	3*	6	<.001	—
Immediate conversion to open repair (%)	7.6	7.1	5.8	NA	—	4.8
Type I endoleaks at discharge (%)	3.3	3.7	7.6	NA	—	3.7

*Compared with controls.

Abbreviations: A-I, Aorto-monoiliac; *FDA,* Food and Drug Administration; *ICU,* intensive care unit; *NS,* not significant; *NA,* not applicable.

pared with the control group. However, this reduction was not sta-
tistically significant for patients receiving A-I endografts who were
at increased risk because of a higher preoperative incidence of myocardial infarction, arrhythmias, and peripheral arterial occlusive
disease. The major decrease in complications occurred in cardiac
and respiratory problems and operative bleeding, whereas renal failure and wound hematoma were more commonly encountered after
endovascular therapy.

Operative blood loss, the requirement for intensive care, and the
duration of postoperative hospital stay were markedly less for all 3
endograft configurations than for SOR patients. With increasing experience and confidence in the procedure, few patients are currently
referred to the intensive care unit, and most are discharged from the
hospital on the first postoperative day.

LONG-TERM RESULTS

Long-term follow-up is essential to compare endovascular management of AAA with SOR and to test the durability of specific devices.
There are no data from prospective randomized trials, and the results from Guidant trials, although prospective, are based on comparisons with concurrently performed open surgery in patients who
did not meet the anatomic criteria for endograft deployment. The
current versions of Ancure tube and bifurcation endografts were initially implanted more than 6 years ago so that enough patient data
are available at this time to provide reliable follow-up to 4 years. A
total of 162 patients with tube endografts were selected for mandatory 5-year follow-up, including all the 153 patients enrolled in
phase 2 and the first 9 patients enrolled in phase 3. For patients with
bifurcation grafts, 268 were from phase 2 and 80 from phase 3 for a
total of 348 patients. All calculations of survival are based on the
intent to treat. Only 1-year follow-up information is available for the
A-I endograft.

The purpose of endograft therapy is to prevent aneurysm rupture. Therefore, the primary outcomes to be considered are patient
survival, the incidence of rupture, and the need for secondary procedures to prevent rupture. In addition, it is important to register
those markers that may lead to failure, which include endoleaks,
aneurysm enlargement, endograft migration, graft occlusion, graft
infection, and loss of endograft integrity.

PATIENT SURVIVAL

There were no significant differences in overall patient survival at 4
years among the tube, bifurcation, and control patient groups (Fig

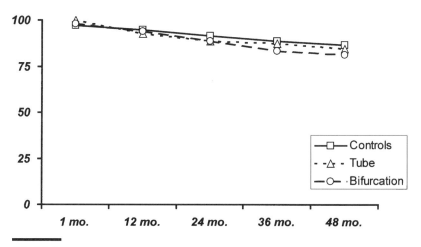

Patient survival

FIGURE 2.

Life-table analysis of patient survival up to 4 years after endograft therapy for the tube and bifurcation implants and standard surgical repair. These curves also represent rupture-free survival, since there were no aneurysm ruptures after endograft implantation among the clinical trial patients who were under long-term surveillance.

2). Deaths occurring more than 1 month after implantation were caused by associated disease problems that were unrelated to the aneurysm, the treatment method, or the vascular prosthesis used. Rupture-free survival was identical to gross survival, since there were no ruptures in either the tube or bifurcation patient groups that were under long-term FDA surveillance. However, a few ruptures, to be described, have occurred among those patients treated since market approval and, therefore, were not in the follow-up cohort for the clinical trials.

At 48 months, the survival without rupture or conversion to SOR for the bifurcation patients (79%), although slightly lower, was not significantly different than survival for the controls (86%). However, it was significantly lower for the tube group (75%, $P < .05$) when compared with controls (Fig 3).

Survival free of rupture, conversion, and other secondary interventions for the tube and bifurcation endografts is presented in Figure 4. Most other secondary interventions were endovascular procedures that were performed to resolve endoleaks in the tube patients or endoleaks and iliac limb obstruction in the bifurcation group.

ANEURYSM RUPTURE

There have been 7 ruptured aneurysms after insertion of endografts of the current, second-generation endograft design. Two patients were treated with tube grafts after market approval and have been previously reported.[5] One developed an endoleak caused by widening of the distal aortic neck that was not recognized because of loss to follow-up for 32 months. The aneurysm was successfully repaired by SOR. The other occurred 6 months after implantation because of an endoleak that resulted from failure to effectively attach the graft in a distal aortic neck that was too wide and lined with thrombus. The patient refused surgery and died.

Five ruptures have occurred in patients treated with bifurcation endografts. One patient had been managed under the phase 3 trial protocol but was not included in the mandated follow-up cohort, and 4 patients received their implants subsequent to market approval. The first occurred in a man with an angulated proximal neck who developed a proximal endoleak that could not be resolved at

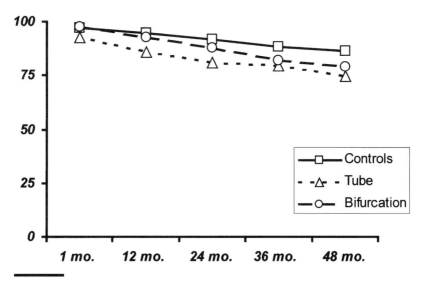

Rupture free survival without conversion

FIGURE 3.

Life-table analysis of patient survival up to 4 years without rupture or conversion to open surgical repair for patients treated with tube and bifurcation endografts compared with controls. The difference at 4 years between the control patients and those treated with tube endografts was significant (86% vs 75%, $P < .05$).

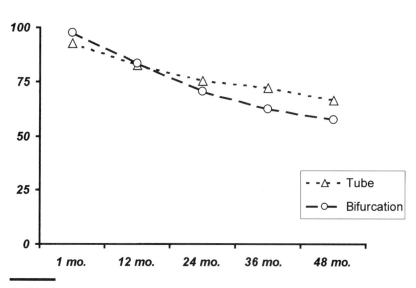

Patient survival without rupture, conversion or other intervention

FIGURE 4

Life-table analysis of survival without rupture, conversion, or other secondary intervention up to 4 years for patients treated with tube and bifurcation endografts. No data were available regarding secondary interventions for the control patients.

the time of implantation. He missed 2 scheduled follow-up appointments and was not seen until rupture occurred 8 months later. The aneurysm was successfully repaired with SOR. In the second patient, prior attempts to treat an iliac attachment endoleak with coils, iliac artery ligation with femoro-femoral bypass, and hypogastric embolization had failed. Rupture occurred 32 months after initial implantation and was successfully treated by coil embolization of the graft limb that was the source of the persistent leak. The third rupture occurred 19 months after implantation and was caused by a type I iliac endoleak that may have been a consequence of prior endovascular instrumentation for a cardiac procedure. This was successfully treated by limited open repair of the leak with an interposition graft between the endograft limb and the distal iliac artery. The fourth was a contained rupture that appeared 1 year after endograft insertion and 6 months after demonstration of a proximal endoleak that was not promptly addressed because of patient delay. This was successfully treated by conversion to open repair. In the fifth patient, rupture appeared 11 months after endograft insertion and was successfully managed by SOR. A short and severely angled proximal aortic neck was the apparent cause of a type I endoleak that could not be closed at the time of implantation. The managing physicians were misled by an erroneous interpretation of the 6-month computed tomography (CT) scan that incorrectly suggested spontaneous closure of the leak.

In all of these cases, there was an underlying type I endoleak that had not been managed promptly or effectively. The delays were the result of failure to recognize abnormal findings on surveillance imaging studies, inadequate patient follow-up, or postponed treatment of a known endoleak. All 6 of the patients who were treated for rupture survived, and the only death occurred in a patient who refused intervention.

ENDOLEAKS

All patients in phase 2 and 3 who are under the FDA-mandated follow-up protocol were evaluated by both contrast CT and color duplex ultrasound (CDU). These studies are performed within 1 month after implantation, at 6 months, and yearly thereafter. An endoleak was registered if it was demonstrated by either one of these studies. The incidence and characterization of endoleaks identified on long term follow-up were based on the findings of an independent radiology core laboratory. Interestingly, the frequency of endoleaks reg-

TABLE 2.

Endoleaks for Each Configuration of the Ancure Endograft (%)

Endograft	Leak Type	<1 mo	12 mo	24 mo	36 mo	48 mo
Tube (n = 150)	I	3.3	1.6	0.0	2.1	1.7
	II	28.0	18.8	14.5	9.6	10.2
	Unk.	10.7	3.8	5.5	6.4	6.8
	Total	42.0	24.2	20.0	18.1	18.7
Bifurcation (n = 300)	I	3.7	3.6	1.5	0.7	1.9
	II	30.3	22.7	17.5	12.7	11.3
	Unk.	7.3	4.5	5.8	4.2	0.0
	Total	41.3	30.8	24.8	17.6	13.2
Aorto-Monoiliac (n = 112)	I	7.6	2.9	—	—	—
	II	31.3	19.0	—	—	—
	Contra iliac	7.2	7.0	—	—	—
	Unk.	9.6	3.0	—	—	—
	Total	55.7	31.9	—	—	—

Abbreviations: Unk., Unknown source of endoleak; *Contra iliac,* contralateral iliac occlusion leak.

Incidence of types of endoleaks over time for all three configurations of Ancure endografts (%)

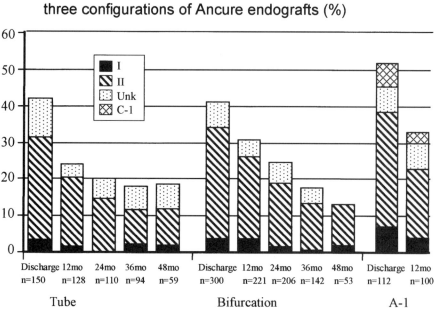

FIGURE 5.

The incidence (%) of types I and II endoleaks and the total percent of patients with endoleaks at yearly intervals from discharge to 4 years for patients with tube and bifurcation endografts. Only 1 year data were available for the aorto-monoiliac (A-I) group. *Abbreviations: Unk,* Unknown source of endoleak; *C-I,* endoleak arising from the contralateral iliac limb occluded by an occlusion device or coils in patients treated with A-I.

istered by the core laboratory was consistently higher than that identified by the investigators.

Table 2 and Figure 5 present the incidence of type I and type II endoleaks and the total number of endoleaks for all 3 endograft configurations. Data beyond 1 year was not available for the A-I endograft system. There have been no type III endoleaks because the unibody construction of Ancure grafts precludes the possibility of modular separation, and there have been no erosions or defects in the polyester graft material.

The incidence of type I endoleaks was low at the time of the initial postimplant study for all 3 graft types and decreased with time in the tube and bifurcation groups followed up to 48 months. This resulted primarily from secondary endovascular interventions to obliterate the leaks with coils, or occasionally by the insertion of a stent or a second endograft. Coil embolization has been highly effective for closing endoleaks and, when successful, is associated with stabilization or shrinkage of the AAA.[6] However, long-term follow-up will be required to determine the ultimate reliability of this technique. Three patients with tube and 3 patients with bifurcation endografts, whose endoleaks failed to respond to endovascular intervention, required late conversions to standard open repair. These were accomplished without operative mortality.

There was a relatively high incidence of type II endoleaks with Ancure devices compared with reports for other endograft designs, and the cause for this difference has not been defined.[7] This may have resulted from the application of CDU in addition to CT for the Ancure trials, whereas only CT was used for the trials of other devices. A recent retrospective study of CT versus CDU noted that the latter was significantly more likely to demonstrate branch leaks than the former, whereas type I leaks were consistently identified by both.[8] The combined use of these imaging modalities may be over-calling the true incidence of branch endoleaks in view of the high rate of AAA shrinkage.[9] Regardless, the incidence of type II leaks diminished with time, and most appeared to have closed spontaneously, since few of these leaks were treated with secondary intervention and none required conversion.

The frequency of type I and II endoleaks in the A-I group was similar to those for the bifurcation and tube patients. However, the higher total in the former reflects the additional leaks at the site of deployment of devices required for contralateral limb occlusion. These were subsequently treated by secondary endovascular procedures. Information regarding the long-term outcome of leaks in patients with this graft configuration is currently unavailable.

CHANGE IN ANEURYSM MORPHOLOGY

Reduction in the size of the aneurysm is a strong indicator that the sac is effectively excluded, and the danger of rupture is eliminated if the AAA does not reexpand. In accordance with the current reporting standards,[10] a change in diameter of 5 mm or more from the postimplant baseline is required to classify an aneurysm as enlarging or diminishing. Half of the aneurysms in the Ancure experience decreased in size within 1 year; this change occurred with all 3 endograft configurations (Fig 6). AAA shrinkage increased to 76.7% at 48 months for patients with bifurcation prostheses, a higher rate than reported for other endograft systems.[11] This is remarkable in view of the high initial incidence of endoleaks. However, most of

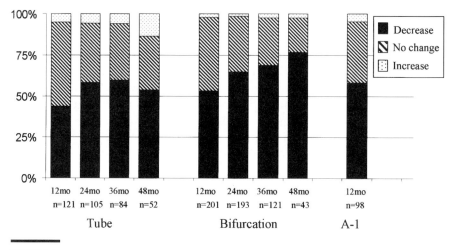

FIGURE 6.

The percentage of patients with a decrease (>5 mm), an increase (>5 mm), or no change (−4.9 to +4.9 mm) in maximum aneurysm diameter from the immediate postimplant baseline to 4 years after implantation of tube and bifurcation grafts. Only 1 year data were available for the aorto-monoiliac *(A-I)* patients.

these were type II leaks that have a tendency to close spontaneously and are infrequently associated with aneurysm expansion.

By contrast, in the patients with tube grafts, the rate of shrinkage did not progress after the first year, and in fact, a small number tended to enlarge after 4 years. The cause for this is not clear but may be related to difficulties in achieving and maintaining graft attachment just above the aortic bifurcation and the known tendency for this segment of the aorta to dilate.[12] Although there was no abrupt appearance of late endoleaks in the tube group, 3 patients with tube grafts manifested increasing AAA diameter in the absence of any demonstrable leak, a situation currently classified as endotension.[10] All 3 patients were successfully managed by conversion to SOR.

Long-term data are not yet available for the A-I endograft system.

REDUCED GRAFT LIMB FLOW

The Ancure endograft is intentionally designed without circumferential or longitudinal support to facilitate endograft deployment in tortuous vessels and to enhance accommodation to changes in aneurysm morphology associated with postimplant shrinkage. As a consequence, the iliac limb of the graft may become obstructed when it is impinged on by atherosclerotic plaques, by kinking when enclosed in a tortuous iliac vessel, or may become redundant when compressed within a small-caliber artery. Evidence for obstruction appeared intraoperatively or developed within the first year in 38% of patients with bifurcation and 30% with A-I endografts. The potential for this problem was often recognized during implantation by the presence of deformities in the completion arteriogram, measurement of differential pressures, or the use of intravascular ultrasound. Thus, among the patients treated for limb obstruction in the first year, 71% were managed at the time of implant. The narrowed segment was usually dilated by balloon angioplasty and placement of a flexible stent, with rare loss of patency during follow-up. A femoro-femoral bypass was required in 6 patients with bifurcation grafts in whom the obstructed area could not be relieved by endovascular techniques, and 3 patients were treated by direct suture anastomosis through a small retroperitoneal incision.

The incidence of graft obstruction in the bifurcation patients was infrequent after the first year. Ten patients developed limb obstruction during the second year of follow-up and 3 patients in the third year. All 13 patients were successfully treated; 9 by endovascular techniques, 2 by femoro-femoral bypass, 1 by retroperitoneal graft limb revision, and 1 by conversion.

Graft limb obstruction appearing at any time after endograft implantation was more commonly caused by stenosis rather than complete thrombotic occlusion. Under the latter circumstances, the graft lumen was restored successfully in most cases by lytic therapy followed by balloon angioplasty and stent placement to eliminate the underlying stenosis.

One patient in the A-I group developed paraparesis after thrombosis of the A-I endograft in the immediate postoperative period. The occlusion was successfully managed by thrombectomy and stent placement, with partial resolution of the neurologic deficit.

The femoro-femoral portion of the A-I has been remarkably durable.[1] Graft thrombosis has not occurred in any of the 114 patients in whom the primary procedure was successfully completed.

GRAFT MIGRATION

Fixation of the proximal aortic attachment site has been remarkably stable for all Ancure configurations, and this appears to be because of the reliability of the hook-bearing attachment system when deployed in a properly sized infrarenal aortic neck. Only one patient developed distal migration at this site. This appeared after 1 year

and eventually produced a proximal endoleak with aneurysm expansion that was successfully treated by conversion 5 years after
implantation. On review of the preoperative CT, it was apparent that
the diameter of the neck in this patient was too large for safe deployment of the endograft.

Proximal migration of the distal aortic attachment system of a
tube endograft developed in 4 patients and produced type I endoleaks. These occurred as a result of dilatation of the distal aortic
neck. All 4 were successfully treated, 3 by the endovascular placement of a bifurcation endograft to bridge the attachment defect, and
the fourth by conversion to SOR.

ENDOGRAFT INTEGRITY

Four-view abdominal X-rays are required to search for fractures of
the metal attachment systems at 3- to 6-month intervals for all patients in the mandated follow-up protocol for all 3 configurations of
the Ancure endograft. Isolated single hook fractures were identified
in 2 patients 3 years after implantation.[13] Each appeared in a proximal attachment system and was not associated with migration or
endoleak. Both patients are asymptomatic, and the diameters of the
aneurysms have decreased. They will continue to be observed under
the standard follow-up protocol, with the intent to convert if migration, endoleak, or aneurysm expansion should appear. There have
been no instances of erosion, tear, perforation, or dilatation of the
fabric of the graft wall.

ENDOGRAFT INFECTION

Infection of the endograft occurred in 2 patients. This complication
appeared after a bout of severe urinary sepsis in one woman who
was residing in a nursing home and was too debilitated for surgical
intervention. She was treated with intravenous and oral antibiotics,
which appeared to have controlled the problem when last evaluated
6 months later. The other patient was treated successfully by graft
excision and axillo-femoral bypass.

DISCUSSION

The operative mortality rate after endograft therapy was equivalent
to that of open aneurysm repair for all 3 configurations of the Ancure
device evaluated in the investigational device exemption trials. This
low rate has been maintained since market approval as noted in the
recently conducted study. The overall 30-day morbidity rate was significantly less than that for open surgical controls. These results are
reflected in a marked reduction in intensive care unit usage, early

discharge from the hospital, and rapid return to preoperative activity levels. Similar early results have been reported for the devices developed by other manufacturers, and these experiences have stimulated an enthusiastic acceptance by patients and their physicians for this less painful and debilitating form of therapy. However, long-term results that are at least equivalent to those of standard surgery are needed to determine whether these early salutary outcomes will be sustained.

The 4-year results for the Ancure tube and bifurcation devices are excellent and suggest that overall survival and survival without rupture are equivalent to standard surgery for that period of observation. Although these outcomes are very encouraging, follow-up data for all patients in the long-term study group for at least 5 years and preferably longer will be required to reliably compare this endograft design with SOR.

Some issues that are unique to endograft therapy for AAA must be considered before we can conclude that endovascular management is an improvement or is at least as effective as SOR. There have been no postimplant AAA ruptures in the phase 2 and 3 clinical trial patients; however, this complication has appeared in 7 patients among the more than 10,000 treated since market approval was granted. Although this appears to be a very infrequent problem, the true incidence of rupture among the postmarket patients cannot be determined because these endograft recipients were not under rigorous investigative surveillance. Furthermore, the average interval between insertion and rupture was 19 months, which is longer than the period since implantation for many of these endografts. All the ruptures were potentially preventable if the prescribed follow-up regimen had been maintained, known endoleaks had been treated in a timely fashion, follow-up imaging had been correctly interpreted, and the anatomic guidelines for case selection had been observed. Fortunately, rupture management was successful in all of the 6 treated patients. These excellent results concur with the report by May et al[14] who suggested that the presence of an endograft protects the patient from the devastating effects of aneurysm rupture. This stands in marked contrast to the poor outcome expected for patients whose aneurysms rupture without prior endograft placement.[15] It is also significantly better than the operative mortality rate of 41% reported in a recent review of published cases of aneurysm rupture after endograft therapy.[5]

The impact of secondary procedures that may be required to treat leaks, graft migration, progressing aneurysm expansion, graft limb obstruction, and endograft infection must be included when evaluating endograft therapy. Among the Ancure-treated patients, the vast majority of these were accomplished by endovascular techniques with low morbidity, no mortality, a high degree of long-term success, and brief hospitalization. Surgical conversion after successful endograft placement was required infrequently and was performed with no operative mortality. The incidence and types of secondary interventions, their physiologic consequences, costs, and patient reactions need to be factored into future studies of devices from each manufacturer to determine the advantage or equivalence of specific endograft designs versus standard surgical management.

All patients treated by endograft exclusion of their aneurysms must be enrolled in a follow-up protocol that includes imaging studies that are expensive and require skilled interpretation of the findings. Both physician commitment and patient acceptance are necessary to ensure that endoleaks, AAA enlargement, endograft migration, or loss of prosthetic integrity are identified and appropriately managed in a timely fashion. The costs and the willingness of patients to comply with these follow-up regimens must also be included in any comparative study.

The use of tube endografts has decreased significantly since completion of enrollment in the clinical trials, and the bifurcation design has been used in more than 96% of patients subsequent to FDA market approval of the Ancure devices. This has occurred because of a concern for reliable fixation of the tube at the aortic bifurcation when the distal aortic neck measurements are marginal, and the known tendency for dilatation of the distal aortic neck. Therefore, Guidant has discontinued the manufacture of the tube device, although this endograft configuration retains FDA market approval.

SUMMARY

All configurations of the Ancure endograft system are initially effective for the endovascular management of infrarenal AAAs, with a low operative mortality rate and a morbidity rate that is less than that of standard surgical repair. The bifurcation device can now be successfully deployed in at least 95% of patients who meet anatomic selection criteria. Patient survival without AAA rupture at 4 years is equal to that of SOR. Although aneurysm rupture has occurred after endograft placement, this has been an infrequent event that is preventable, and all patients who were treated for this complication have survived. Secondary procedures to manage endoleaks, aneurysm enlargement, and graft limb obstruction are required in some patients, but these are usually accomplished by using endovascular methods that are associated with minimal morbidity. Late conversion to SOR, when required, has been performed without operative mortality. Ultimate comparison of open aneurysm repair to endograft exclusion with the Ancure system will require longer-term evaluation.

REFERENCES

1. Rehring TF, Brewster DC, Cambria RP, et al: Utility and reliability of endovascular aortouniiliac graft for aortoiliac aneursymal disease. *J Vasc Surg* 31:1135-1141, 2000.
2. Moore WS, Brewster DC, Bernhard VM: Aorto-uni-iliac endograft for complex aortoiliac aneurysms compared with tube/bifurcation endografts: Results of the EVT/Guidant trials. *J Vasc Surg* 33:S11-S20, 2001.
3. Makaroun MS, Chaikof E, Naslund T, et al: Efficacy of a bifurcated endograft versus open repair of abdominal aortic aneurysms: A reappraisal. *J Vasc Surg* 35:203-210, 2002.
4. FDA Supplement 23 (PMA 990017/S23) Ancure Endograft System. Appendix A. Modifications related to jacket retraction force. Guidant Corporation, May 23, 2001.
5. Bernhard VM, Mitchell RS, Matsumura JS, et al: Ruptured abdominal aortic aneurysm following endovascular repair. *J Vasc Surg* 35:1155-1162, 2002.
6. Amesur NB, Zajko AB, Albert B, et al: Embolotherapy of persistent endoleaks after endovascular repair of abdominal aortic aneurysm with the Ancure-Endovascular Technologies endograft system. *J Vasc Interv Radiol* 10:1175-1182, 1999.
7. Buth J, on behalf of the EUROSTAR Collaborators: Early complications and endoleaks after endovascular abdominal aortic aneurysm repair: Report of a multicenter study. *J Vasc Surg* 31:134-146, 2000.
8. Parent FN, Meier GH, Godziachvili V, et al: The incidence and natural history of type I and II endoleaks: A 5-year follow up assessment by color duplex ultrasound. *J Vasc Surg* 35:474-481, 2002.
9. Makaroun MS: The Ancure endografting system: An update. *J Vasc Surg* 33:S129-S134, 2001.
10. Chaikof EL, Blankensteijn JD, Harris PL, et al: Reporting standards for endovascular aortic aneurysm repair. *J Vasc Surg* 35:1048-1060, 2002.
11. Wolf YG, Hill BB, Rubin GD, et al: Rate of change in the abdominal aortic aneurysm diameter after endovascular repair. *J Vasc Surg* 32:108-115, 2000.
12. Matsumura JS, Chaikof EL: Continued expansion of aortic necks after endovascular repair of abdominal aortic aneurysms. *J Vasc Surg* 28:422-431, 1998.
13. Najibi S, Steinberg J, Katzen BT, et al: Detection of isolate hook fractures 36 months after implantation of the Ancure endograft: A cautionary note. *J Vasc Surg* 34:353-356, 2001.

14. May J, White GJ, Waugh R, et al: Rupture of abdominal aortic aneurysms: A concurrent comparison of outcomes of those occurring after endoluminal repair versus those occurring de novo. *Eur J Vasc Endovasc Surg* 18:344-348, 1999.

15. Heller JA, Weinberg A, Arons R, et al: Two decades of abdominal aortic aneurysm repair: Have we made any progress? *J Vasc Surg* 32:1091-1100, 2000.

CHAPTER 6

Endovascular Abdominal Aortic Aneurysm Repair Using the AneuRx Stent Graft

Christopher K. Zarins, MD
Chidester Professor of Surgery, Chief, Division of Vascular Surgery, Stanford University, Stanford, Calif

Frank R. Arko, MD
Assistant Professor of Surgery, Director of Endovascular Surgery, Division of Vascular Surgery, Stanford University Hospital, Stanford, Calif

Endovascular repair of abdominal aortic aneurysms (AAAs) provides a less-invasive alternative to standard open surgical reconstruction, with reduced morbidity and more rapid patient recovery. During the past 10 years, a number of endovascular devices have been developed with favorable early results.[1-10] The AneuRx stent graft (Medtronic, Santa Rosa, Calif) is one of two Food and Drug Administration (FDA)-approved endovascular devices for the treatment of infrarenal AAAs, with clinical experience now exceeding 5 years. This chapter reviews the current clinical indications, patient selection, and results of treatment with this device.

ANEURX STENT GRAFT

The AneuRx stent graft is a modular, bifurcated endovascular device designed to treat infrarenal aortic and aortoiliac aneurysms.[8] Each stent-graft module consists of a nickel-titanium (Nitinol) exoskeleton joined to a thin-walled noncrimped woven polyester graft. The self-expanding Nitinol stent provides both radial and columnar structural support throughout the length of the stent graft. The primary modular components are a main bifurcated segment and a contralateral iliac limb. Additional modular components include aortic and iliac extender cuffs (Fig 1). Each individual stent-graft module is loaded inside a delivery catheter, which is passed over a stiff 0.035-in guidewire, and positioned by means of angiographic and fluoroscopic control. The self-expanding stent graft is deployed by retraction of the delivery catheter-covering sheath with the use of a deployment handle. The bifurcated device is available in aortic diameter sizes from 20 to 28 mm and passes through a 22F sheath. Iliac diameter sizes range from 12 to 16 mm, and the iliac module

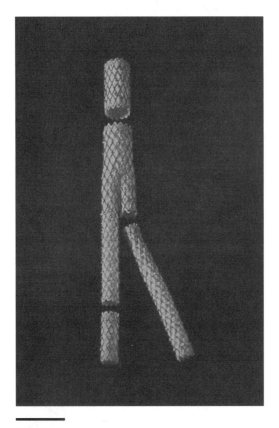

FIGURE 1.

The AneuRx stent graft: a modular, bifurcated endovascular device for the treatment of infrarenal abdominal aortic aneurysms. Each stent-graft module consists of a woven polyester graft joined to a self-expanding Nitinol exoskeleton. Proximal and distal extender modules are used to increase length and secure fixation.

passes through a 16F sheath. The primary bifurcated module is available in lengths of 13.5 cm and 16.5 cm. Length adjustments can be made by using proximal and distal extender cuffs.

PATIENT SELECTION

Indications for endovascular repair of AAAs are no different from open surgical repair and include patients with infrarenal aneurysms 5 cm in diameter or greater, or patients with symptomatic aneurysms. In addition, selected patients with aneurysms between 4 and 5 cm in diameter with a documented increase of 0.5 cm in the past 6 months, and patients with aneurysms twice the diameter of the infrarenal neck may be considered for treatment. However, unlike open surgical repair, specific anatomic criteria must be met for a patient to be a suitable candidate for endovascular repair. For the AneuRx stent graft, these requirements include an infrarenal neck diameter no larger than 26 mm so that appropriate oversizing of the stent graft can be achieved. The largest diameter AneuRx stent graft is 28 mm. Infrarenal neck length should be at least 15 mm in length and without excessive tortuosity, to allow secure proximal fixation of the device. The common iliac arteries should be no larger than 15 mm in diameter for a length of 2 to 3 cm to allow for oversizing and fixation length. Iliac artery tortuosity is an important consideration, as is external iliac diameter, which must be large enough to allow introduction of a 21F delivery catheter on one side and a 16F sheath on the contralateral side. Whereas iliac artery issues of diameter, stenosis, tortuosity, and calcification can often be dealt with by a variety of techniques, patients who have an inadequate infrarenal neck because of diameter, length, or angulation should not be selected for treatment. For example, large-diameter common iliac arteries can be treated by placement of aortic extender cuffs (20-28 mm in diameter, 3.75 cm in length) in a "bell-bottom" configuration. Small-diameter external iliac and common femoral arteries can be accommodated by using 8-mm prosthetic grafts sewn to the external or common iliac arteries and used as conduits to introduce the delivery catheters. Internal iliac arteries can be preserved by bypass or transposition and usually need to be embolized or occluded only when an internal iliac aneurysm is present.

IMAGING

Preoperative imaging is critical for proper patient selection and successful planning for endovascular repair. The most important diagnostic test is a contrast spiral computed tomography (CT) scan with

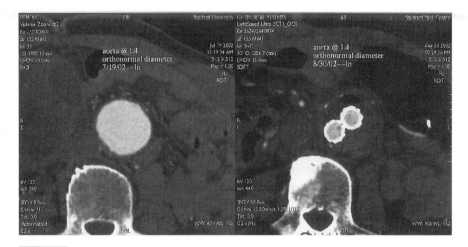

FIGURE 2.

Cross-sectional images of spiral CT scans taken before and after stent graft repair of a 5.5 cm AAA. There is no contrast filling of the aneurysm sac after stent graft placement, indicating complete aneurysm exclusion with no endoleak.

3-mm interval cuts. This is usually performed with a single timed bolus of intravenous contrast (usually 100-120 mL) with scanning of the abdomen and pelvis during a 30-second breath hold. The field of view extends from the diaphragm to the femur, and the contrast bolus is usually delayed 10 to 15 seconds to allow optimal contrast visualization of the abdominal aorta and its branches. The volumetric data can be used to construct 3-dimensional images that are very useful in treatment planning. Similar volumetric 3-dimensional imaging can be performed with gadolinium-enhanced magnetic resonance imaging in patients with compromised renal function.

When high-quality 3-dimensional reconstructions are not available, additional imaging with conventional angiography should be performed to assess the infrarenal aortic neck, identify accessory renal arteries, and evaluate aortic and iliac angulation, tortuosity, and caliber. This should be performed with a 1-cm graduated angiographic catheter with anteroposterior and lateral views. Diameter measurements are best determined by CT with caliper measurements of the outer vessel wall. Angiographic images can be misleading since only the lumen contour is visualized. Length determinations on axial CT can be misleading because of vessel tortuosity. Conventional angiography with a marker catheter or 3-dimensional CT image processing can give better length estimates.

Postoperative imaging should include a postprocedure contrast spiral CT scan to evaluate stent-graft position and aneurysm size, and to determine whether complete aneurysm exclusion has been achieved (endoleak) (Fig 2). Three-dimensional image reconstruction provides useful information on stent-graft position (Fig 3) and allows determination of aneurysm sac volume. In addition, a 2-view plain abdominal x-ray should be obtained to visualize the stent graft. Duplex ultrasound imaging and magnetic resonance imaging are useful in patients with compromised renal function. Postoperative surveillance should be performed at 6- to 12-month intervals for ongoing monitoring and surveillance.

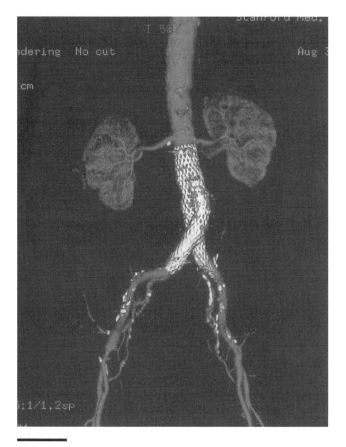

FIGURE 3.

Three-dimensional reconstruction of spiral CT scan demonstrating the stent graft in position below the renal arteries, with complete exclusion of the aortic aneurysm.

TECHNIQUE FOR DEVICE IMPLANTATION

Epidural or general anesthesia may be used with exposure of both common femoral arteries through transverse or vertical groin incisions. These can be extended if iliac exposure is needed. Systemic anticoagulation with heparin is instituted to prolong the activated clotting time to greater than 250 seconds. The activated clotting time is monitored and maintained at this level throughout the procedure, and additional heparin is given as needed.

The femoral arteries are cannulated with an 18-gauge needle, and 0.035-in guidewires are placed bilaterally under fluoroscopic guidance; 10F sheaths are then placed over the 2 guidewires and advanced into the aneurysm under fluoroscopic guidance. A super-stiff 0.035-in guidewire 260 cm in length is inserted into the thoracic aorta, usually from the right limb. In the contralateral iliac artery, a pigtail catheter is placed just above the level of the renal arteries, and an initial roadmapping aortogram is obtained. The 10F sheath in the right femoral artery is exchanged for a 22F sheath, which is placed over the superstiff guidewire and carefully advanced into the proximal infrarenal aorta under fluoroscopic guidance. The main stent-graft module, which is chosen on the basis of preoperative measurements, is then advanced over the guidewire and through the delivery sheath into the perirenal aorta. A second aortogram is performed to verify the position of the renal arteries. Under fluoroscopic guidance, the stent graft is then gradually deployed by retracting the outer sheath and allowing the graft to expand, and it is positioned directly below the level of the renal arteries.

Once the main bifurcation module has been deployed, the 10F sheath in the contralateral iliac artery is pulled back, and a 0.035-in angled hydrophilic wire and a guide catheter are inserted into the contralateral limb of the bifurcation module. The hydrophillic wire is then exchanged for a superstiff guidewire, over which a 16F sheath is advanced into the contralateral limb under fluoroscopic guidance. The contralateral limb is then advanced through the sheath into the contralateral limb and deployed. A final aortogram is then performed to confirm that a satisfactory technical result has been achieved. Proximal and distal extender cuffs may be placed if necessary. The femoral arteriotomies are repaired, and lower extremity perfusion is reestablished.

CLINICAL RESULTS: THE US ANEURX MULTICENTER CLINICAL TRIAL

The AneuRx stent graft was evaluated in a multicenter clinical trial involving 19 US clinical study sites in accord with FDA guidelines.

The first AneuRx device was implanted by Dr Rodney White at Harbor-UCLA on June 3, 1996, initiating the phase 1 feasibility study that involved 40 patients at 4 study sites. The phase 2 controlled study comparing an endovascular-treated group with an open surgical control group was performed at 13 study sites, and the results with 1-year follow-up were presented to the FDA Advisory Panel in June 1999. The phase 3 trial at 19 clinical sites enrolled 641 patients and was concluded when the FDA granted market approval of the device in September 1999. The 4-year results of all 1105 patients in the 3 phases of the trial, along with 87 patients who did not meet the inclusion criteria of the clinical trial and were treated with the AneuRx stent graft on a compassionate use basis during the period of the trial, have been published.[11]

EARLY RESULTS

The initial experience of 190 patients treated with the AneuRx stent graft (both phase 1 and phase 2 patients) was compared with that of 60 surgical control patients with 1-year follow-up, and was presented to the International Society for Cardiovascular Surgery (SCVS) in June 1998 and published in 1999.[1] There were no significant differences in preoperative risk factors of comorbidities between the surgical controls and stent-graft patients. Stent-graft deployment was successful in 97% of patients. There was no difference in operative mortality between the groups (0% in the surgery group and 1% in the stent-graft group). Patients who underwent stent graft repair had 60% less blood loss as compared with patients who underwent open surgery ($P < .001$), and these patients required 80% less blood transfusions ($P < .05$). There was a marked reduction in the time to extubation, discharge from the intensive care unit, ambulation without assistance, and eating a regular diet in the stent-graft group as compared with the surgery group. Major morbidity was reduced by 50% in the stent-graft group ($P < .05$), and hospital length of stay was reduced from 9.3 to 3.4 days ($P < .001$).[1]

PHASE 2 CLINICAL TRIAL

The findings of the phase 2 controlled trial comparing 416 stent-graft patients with 66 patients undergoing open aneurysm repair were presented to the FDA Advisory Panel on June 23, 1999. The results did not differ significantly from the earlier published results and demonstrated the following: successful graft deployment was achieved in 98% of patients, and the surgical conversion rate was 1.5%; there was no difference in the 30-day mortality rate between stent-graft patients (2%) and surgical patients (0%). There was a

50% reduction in major morbidity compared with open repair, a 66% reduction in blood loss, and a 63% reduction in hospital length of stay. Patients recovered more quickly and had earlier return to function compared with patients undergoing open surgery. The physician-reported endoleak rate at the time of hospital discharge was 38%, which was reduced to 13% at 1 month, 16% at 6 months, and 11% at 12 months. Two patients (0.5%) had aneurysm rupture, one during the implantation procedure and one 14 months after implantation of a stiff bifurcation stent graft. These ruptures are included in the later analysis in this chapter.[12] Five percent of patients required a secondary endovascular procedure for endoleak, and 2% required a secondary procedure for nonpatency of the stent graft. Primary graft patency was 98%, and secondary graft patency was 99%.[11]

FOUR-YEAR RESULTS

The 4-year results of all 1192 patients treated during the clinical trial period (1996-1999) with follow-up through June 2000 have been published.[11] The mean follow-up time was 73 months, and there were no patient exclusions for the initial learning curve for device implantation, device design and manufacturing changes, off-protocol compassionate use, or other reasons.

Patients included 1058 men (89%) and 134 women (11%), with a mean age of 73.4 ± 8.0 SD years (range, 45-96 years). Patients had multiple risk factors and comorbidities, and 92% of patients had American Society of Anesthesiologists (ASA) risk classification of III or IV. The mean preoperative aneurysm diameter was 5.6 ± 0.3 SD cm. The mean aneurysm neck length was 27.3 ± 12.2 SD mm, and the mean neck diameter was 22.3 ± 2.9 SD mm. The primary end-point analysis revealed an aneurysm rupture rate of 0.8%, death from aneurysm rupture in 0.3% of patients, death from any cause in 10.3% of patients, early and late surgical conversion (including conversion for rupture) in 2.8% of patients, and a secondary procedure rate for endoleak, migration, or graft nonpatency of 8.0%. The primary graft patency rate was 98%, and the secondary graft patency rate was 99%.

ANEURYSM RUPTURE

The objective of aneurysm repair is to prevent aneurysm rupture and death from rupture. Open surgical repair is generally believed to eliminate the risk of rupture, although there are reports of late ruptures after open repair. Aneurysm ruptures have also been reported after endovascular treatment with each of the various devices thus far evaluated.[12-16] The risk of rupture after treatment with the

AneuRx device is low and appears to be related to adequacy of fixation of the device to the infrarenal neck and iliac arteries.[12] Security of device fixation is influenced by patient selection, precision of device implantation, neck and aneurysm morphology, and changes over time, which may result in device migration. Evidence of insecure fixation can be seen on postimplantation imaging and corrected by placement of extender modules. This is the basis for careful post-procedure imaging and follow-up on a regular basis.

In the early phases of the US clinical trial, a manufacturing change in the primary bifurcation module occurred. The primary bifurcation module initially was manufactured by using a stiff, unsegmented Nitinol stent bifurcation, which was not flexible. This was changed to a segmented Nitinol ring design that resulted in a flexible bifurcation module. The first 174 patients in the clinical trial received the stiff device, whereas the remaining 1018 patients received the flexible design device, which is the current commercial design. The rupture rate for the stiff stent-graft design (6/174) was significantly higher than for the flexible design (4/1018, $P = .002$). Kaplan-Meier analysis revealed freedom from rupture at 3 years in 96% of patients who received the stiff device and 99.5% of patients who received the current design flexible device ($P = .002$). Retrospective analysis of all patients with aneurysm rupture after successful stent-graft repair revealed evidence of insecure fixation of the device either proximally, distally, or at the junction gate, which was identified on imaging studies and potentially could have been treated with stent-graft extender modules, thus possibly avoiding rupture.[11]

ENDOLEAKS

Endoleaks are commonly seen in patients after endovascular aneurysm repair. Although some have considered this to be evidence of an unsuccessful aneurysm repair,[17-21] the true significance of this finding remains unclear.[22,23] We reviewed all patients in phase 2 of the AneuRx clinical trial to determine whether evidence of blood flow in the aneurysm sac (endoleak) was a meaningful predictor of clinical outcome after successful endovascular aneurysm repair. All patients with successful stent-graft implantation and predischarge contrast CT imaging were reviewed by the clinical centers as well as by an independent Core Lab, and the clinical outcome of patients with evidence of endoleak was compared with that of patients without evidence of endoleak.[23] The centers reported endoleaks in 152 of 398 patients (38%) on predischarge CT, whereas the Core Lab reported endoleaks in 50% of these patients ($P < .001$). Follow-up extended to 2 years (mean, 10 ± 4 months) There were no differences between patients with and patients without endoleak before discharge in the following outcome measures: patient survival, aneurysm rupture, surgical conversion, need for a secondary procedure, aneurysm enlargement greater than 5 mm, appearance of a new endoleak, or stent-graft migration. Despite a higher endoleak rate reported by the Core Lab, neither Core Lab-defined endoleaks nor center-defined endoleaks at discharge were significantly related to subsequent outcome measures. The outcome of patients with type I or type II endoleaks before discharge was no different from that of patients without endoleak.[23]

At 1 month, the endoleak rate had decreased to 13%. Although patients with persisting endoleaks were more likely to experience aneurysm enlargement at 1 year, there was no difference in patient survival, aneurysm rupture rate, surgical conversion, new endoleak, or stent-graft migration between patients with and without endoleak at 1 month. Kaplan-Meier survival of all patients undergoing endovascular aneurysm repair was 96% at 1 year and was independent of endoleak status.[23]

Thus, the presence or absence of endoleak on CT scan after AneuRx stent-graft aneurysm repair does not appear to predict long-term outcome. Whereas the identification of blood flow in the aneurysm sac after endovascular repair is a meaningful finding, the usefulness of endoleak as a primary indicator of procedural success or failure remains unproved. Thus, all patients who have undergone endovascular aneurysm repair should be carefully followed up regardless of endoleak status.

COMPARISON WITH OPEN REPAIR

Endovascular repair compares favorably to open surgical repair in the short-term, with a significant reduction in morbidity, reduced blood loss, shorter hospital stay, and earlier return to function.[1,4,9] There was no difference in 1-year patient survival between endovascular and open surgery patients in the phase 2 AneuRx clinical trial. Similarly, concurrent comparison of endoluminal and open repair of aneurysms revealed no differences in survival rate.[24] Long-term controlled trials comparing open with endovascular repair have not yet been reported. Although some have assumed that patients who have undergone open surgical repair are no longer at risk of aneurysm rupture once they have recovered from the operation, this has not proved to be the case. Patients are at risk of pseudoaneurysm rupture, suprarenal and iliac aneurysm formation, graft infection, aortoenteric fistula, and graft thrombosis after open surgical repair.[25-28] The risk of death from late rupture of abdominal aneurysms and pseudoaneurysms after elective open surgical was 5% in 3 large series of 1126 patients followed up for an average of 5 years.[27-30]

Late aneurysm-related deaths after open aneurysm repair, including deaths from ruptured true and false aneurysms, aortoenteric fistula, and graft infections, range from 1.5% to 7.5% in long-term follow-up. Recent reports have also demonstrated that "endoleaks" and ruptures can occur after conventional open aneurysm repair[31] just as they can after endovascular repair. Thus, the true differences in long-term outcome between endovascular and open aneurysm repair remain to be determined. However, the long-term risk of aneurysm rupture after endovascular treatment appears, thus far, to be no higher and perhaps may be lower than after standard open surgical repair.

SUMMARY

The AneuRx stent graft has markedly reduced the morbidity of aortic aneurysm repair and is effective in preventing aneurysm rupture in the great majority of patients. In clinical trial follow-up extending to 4 years, the device is effective in preventing aneurysm rupture in 99.5% of patients. The majority of aneurysm ruptures have occurred in early clinical trial patients who were treated with a stiff bifurcation stent graft, which is no longer manufactured. Thus the long-term risk of rupture may be less than that suggested by early reports. The AneuRx experience suggests that endograft fixation rather than endoleak is the primary determinant of long-term results. Therefore, all patients should be followed up with posttreatment imaging studies to evaluate aneurysm size and stent-graft fixation.

REFERENCES

1. Zarins CK, for the Investigators of the Medtronic AneuRx Multicenter Clinical Trial: AneuRx stent graft vs open surgical repair of abdominal aortic aneurysms multicenter prospective clinical trial. *J Vasc Surg* 29: 292-308, 1999.
2. Becquemin J-P, for the French Vanguard Study Group: Mid-term results of a second-generation bifurcation endovascular graft for abdominal aortic aneurysm repair: The French Vanguard Trial. *J Vasc Surg* 30:209-218, 1999.
3. Brewster DC, Geller SC, Kaufman JA, et al: Initial experience with endovascular aneurysm repair: Comparison of early results with outcome of conventional open repair. *J Vasc Surg* 27:992-1003, 1998.

4. May J, White GH, Weiyun Y, et al: Concurrent comparison of endoluminal versus open repair in the treatment of abdominal aortic aneurysms: Analysis of 303 patients by life table method. *J Vasc Surg* 27:213-221, 1998.

5. Parodi JC, Palmaz JC, Barone HD: Transfemoral intraluminal graft implantation for abdominal aortic aneurysms. *Ann Vasc Surg* 5:491-499, 1991.

6. May J, White GH, Yu W, et al: Importance of graft configuration in outcome of endoluminal aortic aneurysm repair: A five-year analysis by the life table method. *Eur J Endovasc Surg* 15:406-411, 1998.

7. Yusuf SW, Whitaker SC, Chuter TAM, et al: Early results of endovascular aortic aneurysm surgery with aortouniiliac graft, contralateral iliac occlusion, and femorofemoral bypass. *J Vasc Surg* 25:165-172, 1997.

8. White RA, Donayre CE, Walot I, et al: Modular bifurcation endoprosthesis for treatment of abdominal aortic aneurysms. *Ann Surg* 226:381-389, 1997.

9. Moore WS, Rutherford RB: Transfemoral endovascular repair of abdominal aortic aneurysm: Results of the North American EVT phase 1 trial. *J Vasc Surg* 23:543-553, 1996.

10. White GH, Yu W, May J, et al: Three-year experience with the White-Yu endovascular GAD graft for transluminal repair of aortic and iliac aneurysms. *J Endovasc Surg* 4:124-136, 1997.

11. Zarins CK, White RA, Moll FL, et al: The AneuRx stent graft: Four-year results and worldwide experience 2000. *J Vasc Surg* 33:S135-S145, 2001.

12. Zarins CK, White RA, Fogarty TJ: Aneurysm rupture after endovascular repair using the AneuRx stent graft. *J Vasc Surg* 31:960-970, 2000.

13. Lumsden AB, Allen RC, Chaikof EL, et al: Delayed rupture of aortic aneurysms following endovascular stent grafting. *Am J Surg* 170:174-178, 1995.

14. Torsello GB, Klenk E, Kasprzak B, et al: Rupture of abdominal aortic aneurysm previously treated by endovascular stent graft. *J Vasc Surg* 28:184-187, 1998.

15. Alimi YS, Chakfe N, Rivoal E, et al: Rupture of an abdominal aortic aneurysm after endovascular graft placement and aneurysm size reduction. *J Vasc Surg* 28:178-183, 1998.

16. May J, White GH, Waugh R, et al: Rupture of abdominal aortic aneurysms: A concurrent comparison of outcome of those occurring after endoluminal repair versus those occurring *de novo*. *Eur J Vasc Endovasc Surg* 18:344-348, 1999.

17. Schurink GWH, Aarts NJM, va Bockel JH: Endoleak after stent graft treatment of abdominal aortic aneurysm: A meta-analysis of clinical studies. *Br J Surg* 86:581-587, 1999.

18. White GH, Yu W, May J, et al: Endoleak as a complication of endoluminal grafting of abdominal aortic aneurysms: Classification, incidence, diagnosis, and management. *J Endovasc Surg* 41:152-168, 1997.

19. Harris PL: The highs and lows of endovascular aneurysm repair: The first two years of the Eurostar Registry. *Ann R Coll Surg Engl* 81:161-165, 1999.

20. White GH, May J, Waugh RC, et al: Type I and type II endoleaks: A more useful classification for reporting results of endoluminal AAA repair. *J Endovasc Surg* 5:189-193, 1998.

21. Malina M, Ivancev K, Chuter TA, et al: Changing aneurysm morphology after endovascular grafting relation to leakage or persistent perfusion. *J Endovasc Surg* 4:23-30, 1997.

22. Resch T, Ivancev K, Lindh M, et al: Persistent collateral perfusion of the abdominal aneurysm after endovascular repair does not lead to progressive change in aneurysm diameter. *J Vasc Surg* 28:242-249, 1998.

23. Zarins CK, for the AneuRx Clinical Investigators: Endoleak as a predictor of outcome following endovascular aneurysm repair: AneuRx Multicenter Clinical Trial. *J Vasc Surg* 32:90-107, 2000.

24. May J, White GH, Yu W, et al: Concurrent comparison of endoluminal versus open repair in the treatment of abdominal aortic aneurysms: Analysis of 303 patients by life table method. *J Vasc Surg* 27:213-217, 1998.

25. Johnston KW and the Canadian Society for Vascular Surgery Aneurysm Study Group: Nonruptured abdominal aortic aneurysm: Six-year follow up results from the Multicenter Prospective Canadian Aneurysm Study. *J Vasc Surg* 20:163-170, 1994.

26. Cho JS, Gloviczki P, Martelli E, et al: Long-term survival and late complications after repair of ruptured abdominal aortic aneurysm. *J Vasc Surg* 27:813-819, 1998.

27. Rohrer MJ, Cutler BS, Wheeler HB: Long-term survival and quality of life following ruptured abdominal aortic aneurysm. *Arch Surg* 123:1213-1217, 1988.

28. Ruberti U, Scorza R, Biasi GM, et al: Nineteen-year experience on the treatment of aneurysm of the abdominal aorta: A survey of 832 consecutive cases. *J Cardiovasc Surg* 26:547-553, 1985.

29. Crawford ES, Saleh SA, Babb JW III, et al: Infrarenal abdominal aortic aneurysm: Factors influencing survival after operation performed over a 25-year period. *Ann Surg* 193:699-709, 1981.

30. Plate G, Hollier LA, O'Brien P, et al: Recurrent aneurysms and late vascular complications following repair of abdominal aortic aneurysms. *Arch Surg* 120:590-594, 1985.

31. Chan C, Ray SA, Taylor PL, et al: Endoleaks following conventional open abdominal aortic aneurysm repair. *Eur J Vasc Endovasc Surg* 19:313-317, 2000.

CHAPTER 7

Intermediate Results of Endovascular Graft Repair of Abdominal Aortic Aneurysms: The Montefiore Experience*

Takao Ohki, MD
Associate Professor of Surgery and Chief of Vascular Surgery, Montefiore
Medical Center and the Albert Einstein College of Medicine, New
York, NY

Frank J. Veith, MD
Professor of Surgery and Vice President of General Surgery, Montefiore
Medical Center and the Albert Einstein College of Medicine, New
York, NY

A decade has passed since the first endovascular graft (EVG) repair of an abdominal aortic aneurysm (AAA) was performed and reported by Parodi et al.[1] During this period, significant advances have been made in the field. These include the use of EVGs to treat other vascular lesions such as thoracic aneurysms, aortoiliac occlusive disease, iliac aneurysms, vascular trauma, and finally ruptured AAAs. In addition, patient selection and the technology itself have improved markedly. In the early days, the EVGs used were largely surgeon-made devices that required large-caliber delivery systems which made the procedures difficult and risky. In the early 1990s, EVGs were mostly reserved for patients who were deemed

*Supported by grants from the US Public Health Service (HL 02990), the James Hilton Manning and Emma Austin Manning Foundation, the Anna S. Brown Trust, and the New York Institute for Vascular Studies.

high risk for standard surgical repair. When the more sophisticated industry-made EVGs became available, the safety of the procedures improved,[2] and EVGs were also used to treat patients who were good surgical candidates. Since the approval by the Food and Drug Administration (FDA) of the Guidant Ancure graft (Guidant, San Jose, Calif) and the Medtronic AneuRx graft (Medtronic, Inc, Minneapolis, Minn) in 1999, this trend has accelerated further. Currently, the majority of AAAs are treated with EVGs at many hospitals around the world, including our own center. However, the FDA approval was largely based on procedural safety issues, and little long-term proof of efficacy exists to support the widespread use of EVGs, particularly in patients who might be good candidates for a standard open repair.

Recently, a number of investigators reported their midterm results and reached differing conclusions. One positive article was published by May et al.[3] In their analysis, they showed that the long-term patient survival was improved after EVG repair compared with that of patients undergoing open surgery. Zarins et al[4] reported similar encouraging findings. However, a number of other investigators have raised concerns regarding the midterm durability of EVG repair.[5-9] This chapter reviews the intermediate results of EVG repair of AAAs treated at Montefiore Medical Center in New York.

PATIENTS

During the last 10 years, 284 EVG repairs were performed for non-ruptured AAAs. During the same period, 23 ruptured AAAs were treated with EVGs but were excluded from this study.[10] The mean age of the patients was 76 ± 9 years, and 85% were men. The prevalence of associated comorbid conditions including coronary artery disease, chronic obstructive pulmonary disease, diabetes mellitus, hypertension, and chronic renal insufficiency was 86%, 58%, 29%, 86%, and 14%, respectively. The mean American Society of Anesthesiologists (ASA) score was 2.9 ± 0.7, and 80% of the patients had an ASA score of 3 or more.

The mean size of the AAA was 6.2 ± 1.1 cm. The EVGs used were Montefiore EVG or MEGS (105), Ancure/EVT (21), Vanguard (Boston Scientific Corp, Natick, Mass) (16), Talent (World Medical/ Medtronic) (47), Excluder (WL Gore, Flagstaff, Ariz) (20), AneuRx (50), and Zenith (Cook Inc, Indianapolis, Ind) (26). All but the AneuRx and most of the Ancure EVG repairs were performed as part of a phase 1 or phase 2 United States clinical trial under either an investigator or an industry-sponsored Investigational Device Exemption from the FDA.

All patients were followed up with computed tomographic (CT) scans taken 1, 3, 6, and 12 months after the procedure and every 12 months thereafter. Procedural outcomes and follow-up results were prospectively recorded.

DEFINITIONS

- *Technical success* was defined according to the Society for Vascular Surgery/International Society for Cardiovascular Surgery reporting standards as (1) successful EVG deployment without the need for surgical conversion; (2) lack of a persistent (>48 hours) type 1 or type 3 endoleak; and (3) a patent graft.[11]
- *Primary clinical success* was defined as (1) the lack of enlargement of the aneurysm sac (>0.5 cm); (2) the lack of any endoleak (spontaneously sealed endoleaks within 6 months were considered a success); and (3) the lack of the need for any secondary intervention or open surgical procedure. Since we were evaluating the mid- and long-term outcomes, for the purpose of this study, only those patients who survived the operation with a technical success were analyzed by the life-table method.
- *Secondary success* was defined as continued clinical success after a salvage interventional procedure without the need for an open conversion to replace the previously deployed EVG.

TREATMENT METHODS AND STRATEGY FOR ENDOLEAKS

When there was evidence of an endoleak, CT scans were used to determine the type of endoleak. Arteriography was obtained as needed. The basic treatment strategies for various endoleaks are shown in Figure 1.[12] In general, invasive therapy including interventional procedures were reserved for enlarging aneurysms. Stable aneurysms with an endoleak were counted as a clinical failure but were seldom treated. Therapy was also deferred if the patient was a prohibitive risk for any intervention. The treatment strategy depended on the type of endoleak as well as its characteristics.

In summary, short- and large-diameter endoleak channels (mostly types 1 and 3) were treated with either (1) insertion of a second EVG or a proximal or distal cuff (Figs 2 and 3), or (2) surgical conversion. Long- and small-diameter endoleak channels (mostly type 2, some type 1) were treated by inducing thrombosis. This included transarterial and translumbar coil embolization as well as the temporary termination of chronic anticoagulation therapy (Figs 4-6).

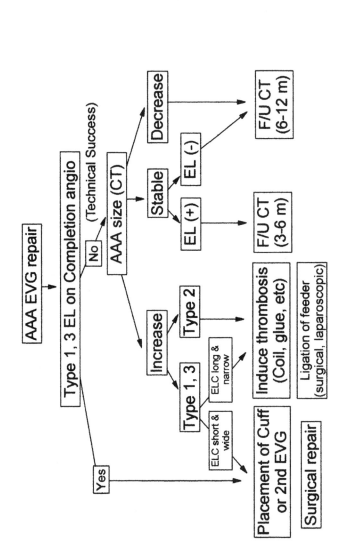

FIGURE 1.

Basic treatment strategy for various endoleaks. *Abbreviations: AAA,* Abdominal aortic aneurysm; *EVG,* endovascular graft; *EL,* endoleak; *angio,* angiography; *CT,* computed tomography; *ELC,* endoleak channel; *F/U,* follow-up. (Courtesy of Ohki T, Veith FJ, Shaw P, et al: Increasing incidence of midterm and long-term complications after endovascular graft repair of abdominal aortic aneurysms: A note of caution based on a 9-year experience. *Ann Surg* 234:323-334, 2001, Lippincott Williams & Wilkins.)

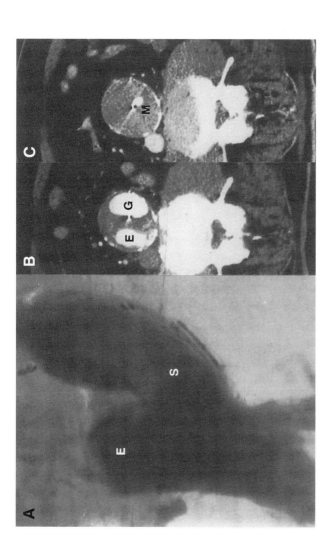

FIGURE 2.

This 80-year-old patient received a tube endovascular graft (EVG) 87 months ago. **A** and **B,** Eighteen months after original EVG *(G)* repair, the patient developed a distal type 1 endoleak *(E).* Since the endoleak channel was short and had a large diameter, inducing thrombosis would not be effective in reducing intrasac pressure, and therefore, a second EVG was needed to exclude the aneurysm. **C,** The Montefiore EVG (MEGS) *(M)* was successfully inserted *via* a femoral approach within the previous EVG, and the endoleak was treated. Eighty-seven months after the initial procedure, the patient continues to do well with continued secondary clinical success. *Abbreviation:* S, Stent. (Courtesy of Ohki T, Veith FJ, Shaw P, et al: Increasing incidence of midterm and long-term complications after endovascular graft repair of abdominal aortic aneurysms: A note of caution based on a 9-year experience. *Ann Surg* 234:323-334, 2001, Lippincott Williams & Wilkins.)

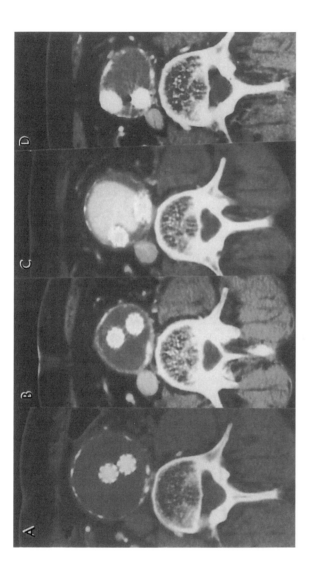

FIGURE 3.

A, Immediate postoperative contrast computed tomography (CT) scan after endovascular graft (EVG) repair. CT shows complete exclusion of the 6-cm abdominal aortic aneurysm (AAA) with no evidence of an endoleak. **B,** Postoperative CT scan (12 months) shows continued exclusion of the AAA with shrinkage of the AAA sac (4 cm). **C,** Postoperative CT scan (21 months) shows an endoleak with an acutely enlarging AAA sac. This endoleak was a type 1 endoleak (distal attachment). This was treated by deploying a second EVG to bridge the defect between the separated limb and the left common iliac artery. **D,** CT scan obtained 52 months after initial EVG repair and 34 months after the secondary intervention. The AAA has shrunk in size without evidence of further endoleak. (Courtesy of Ohki T, Veith FJ, Shaw P, et al: Increasing incidence of midterm and long-term complications after endovascular graft repair of abdominal aortic aneurysms: A note of caution based on a 9-year experience. *Ann Surg* 234:323-334, 2001, Lippincott Williams & Wilkins.)

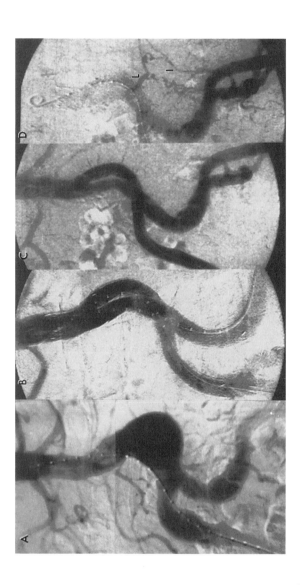

FIGURE 4.

A, Preoperative angiogram reveals the presence of a 5-cm abdominal aortic aneurysm (AAA) with tortuous iliac arteries. **B**, Completion angiogram shows successful exclusion of the AAA with no signs of an endoleak. **C**, The patient developed a late endoleak at 18 months, and a transfemoral angiogram was obtained. Note the lack of endovascular graft migration. **D**, Delayed image of the angiogram reveals a type 2 endoleak arising from the left iliolumbar artery *(I)*, which was feeding the aneurysm via a patent lumbar artery *(L)*. Chronic anticoagulation therapy was terminated for 3 months; however, this endoleak persisted with further enlargement of the AAA. (Courtesy of Ohki T, Veith FJ, Shaw P, et al: Increasing incidence of midterm and long-term complications after endovascular graft repair of abdominal aortic aneurysms: A note of caution based on a 9-year experience. *Ann Surg* 234:323-334, 2001, Lippincott Williams & Wilkins.)

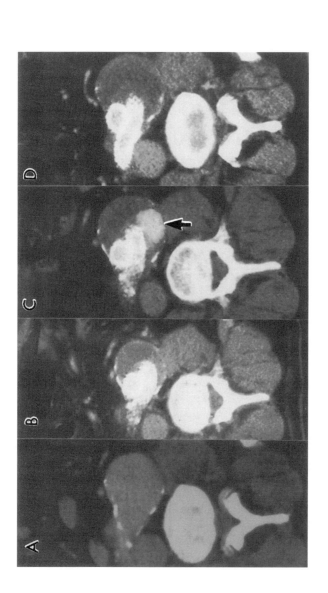

FIGURE 5.

Serial computed tomography (CT) scans of the patient shown in Figure 4. **A,** Preoperative CT shows a 5-cm abdominal aortic aneurysm (AAA). **B,** Six months after endovascular graft repair. An endoleak is not visualized, and the AAA has shrunk in size. **C,** CT scan after 12 months shows the presence of an endoleak and an enlarging AAA (5.5 cm). **D,** CT scan obtained 20 months after translumbar coil embolization (Fig 6). The endoleak has resolved. This patient continues to do well 36 months postoperatively. (Courtesy of Ohki T, Veith FJ, Shaw P, et al: Increasing incidence of midterm and long-term complications after endovascular graft repair of abdominal aortic aneurysms: A note of caution based on a 9-year experience. *Ann Surg* 234:323–334, 2001, Lippincott Williams & Wilkins.)

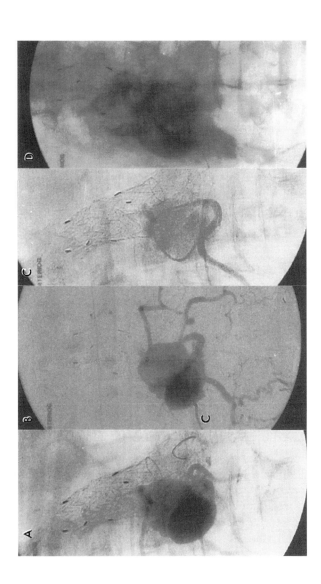

FIGURE 6.

A and **B**, Since conservative therapy failed (Fig 4, D), translumbar puncture of the sac was performed. Sac-gram reveals the presence of multiple feeding arteries in addition to the iliolumbar artery that was depicted by the standard angiogram in Figure 4, D. Sac pressure was equivalent to systemic blood pressure (*c*, translumbar catheter). **C**, Selective coil embolization of all 4 lumbar arteries was performed. **D**, Completion sac-gram shows lack of communication between the lumbar arteries and the abdominal aortic aneurysm (AAA) sac, and the contrast is stagnant in the isolated AAA. The AAA sac pressure measured 40 mm Hg on completing the selective coil embolization. (Courtesy of Ohki T, Veith FJ, Shaw P, et al: Increasing incidence of midterm and long-term complications after endovascular graft repair of abdominal aortic aneurysms: A note of caution based on a 9-year experience. *Ann Surg* 234:323-334, 2001, Lippincott Williams & Wilkins.)

TREATMENT METHODS FOR OTHER LATE FAILURES

Failing EVGs detected during physical examination or during routine duplex scans were confirmed arteriographically. Percutaneous balloon angioplasty and stenting were preferentially performed for graft narrowing or kinking. Thrombolysis or thrombectomy via an open femoral arteriotomy was performed when the EVG or one limb of it had completely thrombosed. After removal of the clot, an effort was made to correct the underlying defect by stenting. If this proved impossible, an extra-anatomical bypass was performed. The diagnosis of graft infection, including aortoenteric fistula, was made by information derived from multiple tests including physical examination, endoscopy, blood cultures, white blood cell counts, CT, and duplex scans. Treatment was by open conversion or operative drainage (Table 1).

RESULTS

The mean operating room time for the initial EVG placement procedure was 5.4 ± 0.31 hours (range, 1.5-14.1 hours), and the mean blood loss was 120 ± 30 mL. Twenty-three percent of the patients required a homologous blood transfusion. The mean length of stay was 3.9 ± 3.5 days.

The major morbidity and mortality rates within 30 days of EVG repair were 15.6% and 7.4%, respectively. The technical success rate (complete AAA exclusion without perioperative mortality) was 90%. During follow-up to 87 months (mean, 18.7 months), 60 patients (21%) died of unrelated causes. The overall life-table patient survival rate at 5 years was 42%. Sixteen patients (6.3%) were lost to follow-up despite multiple attempts to contact the patient, the family, or their primary medical doctor. During this period, only 2 patients had an aneurysm rupture. Of the patients with AAA rupture, one had been lost to follow-up, and the other had known graft migration, a proximal type 1 endoleak, and an enlarging aneurysm. The aneurysm ruptured while the patient was awaiting a secondary open repair; however, an emergent open repair was performed and the patient survived.

Other late complications included type 1 endoleak (8); aortoduodenal fistula (2), one with an abdominal abscess; graft thrombosis/stenosis (9); limb separation or fabric tear with a subsequent type 3 endoleak (1); and a persistent type 2 endoleak (16). A secondary intervention or open surgical procedure was required in 32 cases (11%) (Table 1). These included deployment of a second EVG (4), open AAA repair (6), transarterial coil embolization (3), translum-

TABLE 1.
Details of the Secondary Procedures

Case No.	Late Complication	Time to Failure (mo)	Presenting Symptom or Study	Secondary Procedure	Outcome	LOS (d)
1	Type 1 leak	21	CT	Open conversion	Success	5
2	Type 1 leak	28	CT	Open conversion	Success	5
3	Type 1 leak/rupture	38	Back pain, CT	Open conversion	Success	5
4	Type 1 leak/rupture	55	Shock, CT	Open conversion	Death	NA
5	Type 1 leak	24	CT	Open conversion	Success	7
6	AE fistula with abscess	9	GI bleed, CT	Open conversion	Death	NA
7	AE fistula	30	Sepsis, CT	Transabdominal drainage	Death	NA
8	Graft thrombosis	1	Foot, rest pain	Axfem bypass	Success	3
9	Graft thrombosis	3	Foot, rest pain	Axfem bypass	Success	3
10	Graft thrombosis	24	Claudication	Axfem bypass	Success	2
11	Graft thrombosis	6	Claudication	Femfem bypass	Success	1
12	Graft thrombosis	8	Rest pain	Femfem bypass	Success	2
13	Graft thrombosis	1	Claudication	Femfem bypass	Success	2
14	Type 1 leak	16	CT	2nd EVG	Success	2
15	Type 1 leak	20	CT	2nd EVG	Success	3
16	Type 1 leak	21	CT	2nd EVG	Success	1
17	Type 3 leak	29	CT	2nd EVG	Success	1
18	Graft thrombosis	10	Leg weakness	Thrombectomy, stent	Success	2
19	Right EIA stenosis	7	Claudication	Thrombectomy, stent	Success	2
20	Left iliac stenosis	6	Claudication	PTA, stent	Success	1
21-23	Type 2 leak	6-29	CT	TFA	2/3 Success	1-2
24-32	Type 2 leak	3-32	CT	TLA	10/11 Success	1-2

Abbreviations: LOS, Length of stay; *CT,* computed tomography; *NA,* not applicable; *AE,* aortoenteric;; *GI,* gastrointestinal; *Axfem,* axillofemoral; *Femfem,* femorofemoral; *EVG,* endovascular graft; *EIA,* external iliac artery; *PTA,* percutaneous transluminal angioplasty; *TFA,* transfemoral coil embolization; *TLA,* translumbar coil embolization.

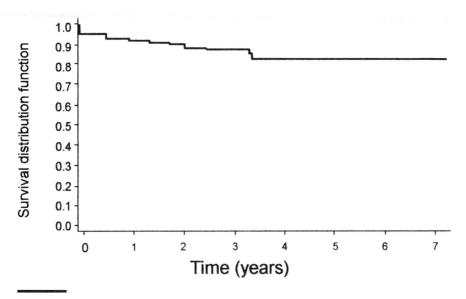

FIGURE 7.

Kaplan-Meier analysis of continued primary clinical success. Success rates (number at risk) at 1, 3, and 5 years were 92% (190), 84% (54), and 84% (10), respectively.

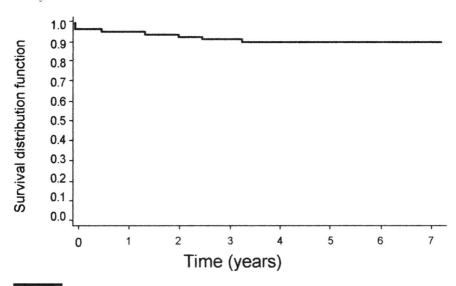

FIGURE 8.

Kaplan-Meier analysis of continued secondary clinical success. Success rates (number at risk) at 1, 3, and 5 years were 95% (210), 92% (56), and 92% (12), respectively.

bar coil embolization (9), extra-anatomical bypass (6), and stent placement (3). The technical success of the nonoperative secondary interventions was 89%, and the mean length of hospital stay for these secondary procedures was 1.3 days. Continued clinical success (Fig 7) and assisted clinical success (Fig 8) are shown with the use of life-table analyses.

COMMENTS

LATE FAILURE IS NOT NECESSARILY A DEFEAT

Recently, a number of investigators have reported their midterm results with mixed conclusions. One favorable article was published by May et al.[3] In their analysis, they showed that the long-term patient survival was better during a follow-up period up to 5 years after EVG repair than it was after open surgical repair in a control group of patients. Zarins et al[4] reported an encouraging rupture-free rate of 99.5% at 3 years with the AneuRx graft. There have been similar encouraging reports on the outcome of the Ancure graft as well.[13] However, a number of others have raised concerns regarding the midterm durability of EVG repair. Zarins himself and his colleagues[14] reported 7 unexpected AAA ruptures after EVG repair, with 5 deaths. Furthermore, the European collaborators reported their experience with 2464 EVGs during a 4-year period. Of these, 14 patients had aneurysm rupture 0 to 24 months after EVG repair, with 9 deaths.[6] Hölzenbein et al[9] reported that 26% of their patients needed to undergo a secondary procedure to treat EVG-related complications during a follow-up period of 18 months. Others reported similar results and raised similar concerns.[7,8]

Our results expand on these findings and concerns.[5] In our series, the procedural time and blood loss, as well as the perioperative mortality rate (7.4%), were higher than in most other reports. This is probably because most (80%) of our patients were elderly high-risk patients, many of whom had large, complex AAAs. In addition, many of our patients had previously been denied both open and EVG repair by other surgeons because of medical comorbidities, aortoiliac anatomic complexity, or both. This made our patient cohort unusually challenging. Even in this difficult group of patients, our technical success rate was high, and perioperative complications, length of hospital stay, and estimated blood loss were reasonably and acceptably low. Nevertheless, the increasing occurrence of late failure with time in our patients whose treatment was originally successful for more than 1 year is alarming. In this regard, it is worth noting that FDA approval of these devices was made based on a fol-

low-up period of only 12 months. Our observation of frequent problems developing after 1 year is consistent with the findings of others.[4,6-9] From our and others' experience, it is clear that EVG repair
is not as durable as open surgical repair. EVGs can fail in a greater
number of ways and with greater frequency than standard AAA
grafts placed at an open operation. These modes of EVG failure included occurrence of late endoleaks, graft thrombosis, aortoenteric
fistulas, and ultimately rupture of the aneurysm with and sometimes without a known endoleak.

Such disadvantages of EVG repair must be weighed against several positive attributes. These include the low mortality rate, even in
patients at high risk for open surgery, and the short length of hospital stay. In addition, it is encouraging that only 2 of our patients had
an aneurysm rupture during the entire study period. Of our patients
that were not lost to follow-up, none had an aneurysm rupture without a preceding known endoleak. That most late failures can be detected before causing a catastrophic event or death is a positive finding. This allows secondary salvage procedures to be performed in a
timely fashion to prevent aneurysm rupture or limb loss. Moreover,
the secondary procedures when required were mostly minimally invasive, and the technical success rate was high (Table 1). Most of the
late problems that we encountered could be treated with percutaneous procedures, and many were done transfemorally. Therefore, late
failure in itself does not necessarily produce a bad overall outcome.
Others have also reported successful outcomes after secondary interventions for late EVG failures.[7,9] On the other hand, failure to detect late failure can lead to aneurysm rupture and death.[6,7,14] Therefore, diligent postoperative surveillance is critically important after
an EVG repair.

ROLE OF EVGS IN CURRENT PRACTICE

At Montefiore Medical Center, approximately 65% of all AAAs were
treated with an EVG during 1997-2000. In 2002, this percentage decreased to 55% as a result of increasing concern regarding long-term
durability. Interestingly, despite the increased concern, more than
half of the patients are still treated with EVGs. This is because of
several factors. First is the presence of nonsurgical candidates. For
those patients who have large or symptomatic AAAs with severe
comorbid conditions precluding open surgery, EVG repair continues to serve as the treatment of choice, and the concern regarding
long-term durability has not affected its use in this group of patients.
Similarly, for those with ruptured AAAs, EVG repair is offered as the
first-line treatment option.[10]

For those patients who are otherwise healthy and have a low surgical risk and whose anatomic characteristics are not favorable for EVG repair, the decision is relatively simple, and open surgery is performed in most instances.

The more difficult question is related to the role of EVGs in the treatment of patients who are good candidates for both an open repair and EVG repair from both an anatomic and medical standpoint. An example of such a patient is a 65-year-old healthy man who has a 6-cm AAA with a well-defined proximal and distal landing zone with good access vessels. In this case, the mortality rate for both open and EVG repair is insignificant, and there is no apparent difference between the two. The difference is in the morbidity rate, period to recuperation, postoperative quality of life, and the long-term durability. EVG repair provides upfront benefit through low morbidity, rapid recovery, and good quality of life, whereas the open repair provides more definitive cure. The treatment of choice under this circumstance depends on how one weighs these factors, and this is not a purely medical decision. If this patient was sexually active and wished to maintain his activity at the expense of undergoing lifelong surveillance with the understanding that he may need a secondary procedure, it is a sound decision. Good-risk patients should be given a choice between an open operation and an EVG repair. Indeed, patients may be encouraged to view the 2 treatment options—standard surgical repair and EVG repair—as the choice between one big operation or the possibility of several smaller operations. However, it must be noted that open surgical repair is also not a perfectly durable operation. In addition to the higher perioperative morbidity rate, graft infection, para-anastomotic aneurysm formation, and graft thrombosis occur after open repair, although the incidence appears to be lower than after EVG repair.[15] Moreover, durability is but one important aspect of the procedure and will not alone determine the superiority of one approach over another. Whether one chooses an EVG repair, which provides early benefit because of its minimally invasive nature, at the cost of possibly undergoing a secondary procedure, or whether one undergoes a single, more definitive but more invasive procedure will depend not only on the results of prospective comparative studies but also on patient preference.

EVG REPAIR: A FAILED EXPERIMENT OR AN INNOVATION IN EVOLUTION

A recent editorial in the *British Journal of Surgery*, entitled "Endovascular Treatment of Abdominal Aortic Aneurysm: A Failed Experiment," makes some worthy points,[16] but we disagree on several points. The authors correctly point out the low rupture rate of small AAAs (<1% per year). They also note the increasing device and procedural failures with time, the preponderance of small AAAs in most EVG series, and the glaring lack of universal follow-up and audited reporting of late results. They indicate that the smaller AAAs which are usually treated by EVGs are those that may be easiest to repair by conventional open surgery. They summarize the appreciable early and late complication rates of EVG repair, and the reintervention and conversion rates. They also note that the rupture risk of 1% per year after EVG repair is not greatly different from the natural history of most of the small AAAs so treated. They conclude by enumerating the forces promoting the rapid adoption of EVGs by surgeons and others—namely, the desire to obtain personal and institutional prestige, and financial gains for surgeons and device manufacturers.

Within the context of their review, some of their points are correct, and surgeons using EVGs should pay them heed. We agree that EVGs should not generally be used to treat AAAs less than 5.5 cm in diameter unless the AAA is clearly enlarging or symptomatic. However, we cannot accept the editorial's conclusion that EVG repair is "a failed experiment." This conclusion would suggest the abandonment of EVG repair. The history of surgical innovation is based on progress through the development of new technology and the selection of appropriate patients. Just because an innovation is imperfect or has risks does not mean it should be abandoned. EVGs will eventually prove to have value in selected (but not all) patients. Better devices and improved patient selection will almost certainly lead to improved results. Thus, EVG repair is certainly here to stay, even though its precise role remains to be defined. We believe that EVG repair is not a failed experiment; it is an innovation in evolution and under evaluation.[17]

CONCLUSIONS

EVG repair is not as durable as open repair. However, the secondary interventions required are relatively minimally invasive procedures with high success rates. Therefore, the need for a secondary intervention does not necessarily represent a failure. Patients need to be informed of the need for lifelong surveillance and the possible need for secondary procedures. For good surgical risk patients, EVG repair should currently be performed with caution and restraint.

REFERENCES

1. Parodi JC, Palmaz JC, Barone HD: Transfemoral intraluminal graft implantation for abdominal aortic aneurysms. *Ann Vasc Surg* 5:491-499, 1991.
2. Zarins CK, White RA, Schwarten D, et al: AneuRx stent graft versus open surgical repair of abdominal aortic aneurysms: multicenter prospective clinical trial. *J Vasc Surg* 29:292-308, 1999.
3. May J, White GH, Waugh R, et al: Improved survival after endoluminal repair with second-generation prostheses compared with open repair in the treatment of abdominal aortic aneurysms: A 5-year concurrent comparison using life table method. *J Vasc Surg* 33:21-26, 2001.
4. Zarins CK, White RA, Moll FL, et al: The AneuRx stent graft: Four-year results and worldwide experience 2000. *J Vasc Surg* 33:135-145, 2001.
5. Ohki T, Veith FJ, Shaw P, et al: Increasing incidence of midterm and long-term complications after endovascular graft repair of abdominal aortic aneurysms: A note of caution based on a 9-year experience. *Ann Surg* 234:323-334, 2001.
6. Harris PL, Vallabhaneni SR, Desgranges P, et al: Incidence and risk factors of late rupture, conversion, and death after endovascular repair of infrarenal aortic aneurysms: The EUROSTAR experience. European Collaborators on Stent/Graft Techniques for Aortic Aneurysm Repair. *J Vasc Surg* 32:739-749, 2000.
7. Marrewijk C, Buth J, Harris PL, et al: Significance of endoleaks after endovascular repair of abdominal aortic aneurysms: The EUROSTAR experience. *J Vasc Surg* 35:461-473, 2002.
8. Bush RL, Lumsden AB, Dodson TF, et al: Mid-term results after endovascular repair of the abdominal aortic aneurysm. *J Vasc Surg* 33:70-76, 2001.
9. Hölzenbein TJ, Kretschmer G, Thurnher S, et al: Midterm durability of abdominal aortic aneurysm endograft repair: A word of caution. *J Vasc Surg* 33:46-54, 2001.
10. Ohki T, Veith FJ: Endovascular grafts and other image guided catheter based adjuncts to improve the treatment of ruptured aortoiliac aneurysms. *Ann Surg* 232:466-479, 2000.
11. Ahn SS, Rutherford RB, Johnston KW, et al: Reporting standards for infrarenal endovascular abdominal aortic aneurysm repair. Ad Hoc Committee for Standardized Reporting Practices in Vascular Surgery of The Society for Vascular Surgery/International Society for Cardiovascular Surgery. *J Vasc Surg* 25:405-410, 1997.
12. Ohki T, Veith FJ: Management of the various types of endoleaks, in Whittemore AD, Bandyk DF, Cronenwett JL, et al (eds): Advances in Vascular Surgery, vol 9. St Louis, Mosby, 2001.
13. Moore WS, Kashyap VS, Vescera CL, et al: Abdominal aortic aneurysm: A 6-year comparison of endovascular versus transabdominal repair. *Ann Surg* 230:298-308, 1999.

14. Zarins CK, White RA, Fogarty TJ. Aneurysm rupture after endovascular repair using the AneuRx stent graft. *J Vasc Surg* 31:960-970, 2000.

15. Hallett JW Jr, Marshall DM, Petterson TM, et al: Graft-related complications after abdominal aortic aneurysm repair: Reassurance from a 36-year population-based experience. *J Vasc Surg* 25:277-284, 1997.

16. Collin J, Murie JA: Endovascular treatment of abdominal aortic aneurysm: A failed experiment (editorial). *Br J Surg* 88:1281-1282, 2001.

17. Veith FJ, Johnston KW: Endovascular treatment of abdominal aortic aneurysms: An innovation in evolution and under evaluation. *J Vasc Surg* 35:183, 2002.

CHAPTER 8

Complications Associated With Endovascular Repair of Abdominal Aortic Aneurysm

Thomas T. Terramani, MD
Resident in General Vascular Surgery, Division of General Vascular
Surgery, Emory University School of Medicine, Atlanta, Ga

William Brinkman, MD
Resident in General Vascular Surgery, Division of General Vascular
Surgery, Emory University School of Medicine, Atlanta, Ga

Sasan Najibi, MD
Resident in General Vascular Surgery, Division of General Vascular
Surgery, Emory University School of Medicine, Atlanta, Ga

Elliot L. Chaikof, MD, PhD
Professor of Surgery, Division of General Vascular Surgery, Emory
University School of Medicine, Atlanta, Ga

Numerous reports have emphasized the benefits of endovascular repair of abdominal aortic aneurysms (AAAs), including an observed decrease in the duration of hospitalization, intensive care unit requirement, and blood loss.[1-3] However, of particular significance has been a perceived reduction in the incidence and magnitude of in-hospital complications, especially among patients at high risk for surgical intervention because of significant comorbidities. For example, in a recent review of open aortic surgery performed on 856 patients at our institution, we observed a major complication rate of 16%.[4] Although a very similar incidence of overall complications was observed in our experience with 236 patients who underwent endovascular AAA repair, complications in this series were characteristically minor, such as superficial wound infections, all of which were successfully treated on an outpatient basis.[5] Otherwise, major morbidity occurred in less than 5% of patients, with 2 episodes of renal failure and 3 cases of myocardial ischemia.

Despite the advantages of endovascular therapy and its acknowledged capacity to reduce major in-hospital morbidity, initial success rates continue to be compromised for those patients that exhibit challenging anatomic states. For example, although a variety of maneuvers have been described to facilitate management of those aneurysms with an inadequate aortic neck or enlarged common iliac arteries, these approaches are not entirely risk-free. Moreover, the ability to achieve a durable outcome, without risk of aneurysm rupture, remains limited among all patients by a variety of problems, including endoleak, endograft durability, and aortoiliac remodeling. Although catastrophic complications of endovascular grafting have included device infection and the formation of aortoenteric fistula, this chapter has as its primary focus those major problems that remain, all too often, a part of the day-to-day practice of endovascular aneurysm repair.

DEPLOYMENT-RELATED COMPLICATIONS

Most reports estimate that the proportion of patients who are suitable for treatment with available commercial endoprostheses ranges between 20% and 50%. Reductions in device profile, enhanced endograft flexibility, and improvements in endograft design to accommodate a wide range of aortic neck and iliac artery diameters will undoubtedly increase the proportion of patients who can be appropriately treated with endovascular grafts. Nonetheless, even among those patients who can be adequately treated with the current generation of commercially available endoprostheses, a variety of adjunctive maneuvers are often required for many aneurysms that would otherwise not be anatomically suitable for endovascular repair. Concomitant procedures to facilitate aneurysm access, such as the use of a brachiofemoral wire or an iliac conduit, can generally be performed with minimal added morbidity.[6,7] However, hypogastric artery (HA) embolization has been the focus of a number of recent investigations because of the potential of significant perioperative morbidity. In particular, whereas embolization of the HA can be conducted in many cases without adverse effects, there remains a finite risk of buttock claudication, and although infrequent, more severe pelvic ischemic syndromes have been noted.

Approximately 20% of patients with AAA have concurrent iliac artery aneurysms.[8] As such, the exclusion of concurrent common iliac artery (CIA) aneurysms sometimes requires the exclusion of the HA to obtain adequate distal attachment of the endograft in the external iliac artery. Similarly, embolization is required if a concurrent HA aneurysm exists. In a reassuring report, Mehta et al[9] reviewed their experience with unilateral HA interruption in 99 patients and 8 cases of bilateral interruption. No instances of buttock necrosis, ischemic colitis requiring laparotomy, or deaths were observed. Although the proximal placement of embolization coils assists in the preservation of critical collateral pathways, approximately 1 in 6 patients did complain of buttock claudication, with symptoms persisting in one third of the patients at 1-year follow-up. The incidence of impotence and minor neurologic deficit was less than 10%. Similar findings have been reported by Lee et al.[10] In our experience, colon and sacral ischemia can occur with acute embolization of both HAs. We believe that staged embolization along with preservation of femoral circumflex vessels reduces the risk of adverse events. However, the suitability of even unilateral HA embolization should be questioned for those patients with a prior history of left colectomy and compromised contralateral pelvic circulation.

IMPLANT-RELATED COMPLICATIONS

With appropriate patient selection, an experienced clinician can anticipate the successful deployment of an endograft in nearly all patients, with most recent reports from high-volume centers noting deployment success rates exceeding 95%. However, the mere presence of a deployed device does not necessarily prohibit aneurysm rupture and death, nor does it preclude the development of other late device-related complications. Indeed, a continuing limitation of endovascular therapy has been the necessity for lifelong surveillance and a requirement for secondary transcatheter or surgical procedures to achieve and maintain a durable outcome. Current estimates suggest that the annual reintervention rate may be as high as 10%.[11-14] In this regard, although graft limb stenosis or thrombosis has been a well-documented complication typically caused by late aortoiliac remodeling, most secondary interventions have been prompted by the presence of a persistent endoleak with or without aneurysm expansion. The potential role of endograft migration and frank device failure as contributing factors in the failure of endovascular therapy is particularly worrisome.

ENDOGRAFT LIMB STENOSIS AND OBSTRUCTION

In general, the development of late graft limb stenosis leading to endograft thrombosis is much more common among unsupported endoprostheses, such as the Ancure endograft (Guidant, Menlo Park, Calif). For example, Baum et al[15] observed that limb kinking requiring reintervention occurred in 44% of unsupported graft limbs, but in only 5% of limbs in patients receiving supported endografts. We have observed that late limb thrombosis may occur 2 or more years after initial endograft placement and often without the development of initial claudication symptoms. As a consequence, in our own unit, we have had a low threshold for the placement of self-expanding stents (Wallstent; Boston Scientific, Natick, Mass) in the limbs of Ancure endografts, particularly if there exists a significant size mismatch between limb and iliac artery diameters. Moreover, the development of significant angulation in an unsupported limb, as viewed on follow-up abdominal radiographs, should prompt angiographic evaluation, even in the absence of symptoms or change in ankle-brachial index. Whereas angioplasty and stenting with or without thrombolysis are useful endovascular options for treatment of the occluded or stenotic limb, a femoro-femoral bypass may be required.

LOSS OF ENDOGRAFT INTEGRITY

Despite rigorous premarketing fatigue testing of endografts, reports of structural failure persist, including fractures of Nitinol frames, Elgiloy hooks, and disruption of endograft fabric. We have recently identified isolated Elgiloy hook fractures in 2 patients 36 months after implantation of a Food and Drug Administration (FDA)-approved Ancure endograft and in an additional patient after the publication of our initial report.[16] Notably, hook fractures were not visualized on all abdominal radiographs, nor were they noted on the institutional report by the reviewing radiologist. Thus, this experience emphasizes that multiple-view abdominal x-rays remain essential for all patients treated with an endograft, with particular attention directed to the integrity of the metal components. Although clinical sequelae were not associated with these hooks fractures, continued vigilance is clearly mandated because of a risk of late endoleak and graft migration. Likewise, Matsumura et al[17] observed the disruption of fixation sutures with the development of fabric "microleaks" in an initial version of the AneuRx graft (Medtronics, Santa Rosa, Calif). The Vanguard endograft (Boston Scientific) unfortunately provides an additional example of an inadequately engineered device, which was withdrawn from clinical studies because of fractures of the Nitinol frame that were occasionally associated with disruption of the endograft fabric.[18] Of some concern have been recent reports of Nitinol corrosion with pitlike surface damage, as well as the presence of stress cracks.[19] The clinical significance of this observation remains to be defined.

ENDOGRAFT MIGRATION

Since the initial observation of gradual dilation of the proximal infrarenal aortic neck, the very real potential of late endograft migration has been recognized.[20] It is of interest that neck expansion has been observed in association with different attachment systems, and consequently, the contribution of device design to this particular problem is unknown.[13,21,22] Although some disagreement exists, clear correlations have not always been demonstrated between neck enlargement and preoperative neck diameter, endograft oversizing, endoleak, or aneurysm size. Cao et al[22] reported a 15% incidence of device migration (>10 mm) among 113 patients treated with AneuRx endografts, nearly half of whom underwent a secondary procedure including either placement of proximal aortic cuffs or conversion to open surgery. Although endograft migration can often follow neck expansion, it is also evident that this complication may also occur because of improper initial patient selection in which the neck is simply too short or wide for the selected device. However, Conners et al[23] have recently emphasized that oversizing of endografts does not necessarily preclude device migration, even in the short-term. In their series, 40% of all AneuRx endografts migrated 5 mm or more, 3 years after initial device implantation. Thirty percent of these patients required a secondary endovascular procedure.

ENDOLEAKS, ENDOTENSION, AND THE RISK OF ANEURYSM RUPTURE

An endoleak may be caused by an incomplete "seal" at either proximal or distal portions of an endograft (type I), by retrograde blood flow from aortic side branches (type II), by an inadequate connection between components of a modular prosthesis (type III), or by direct fabric defects (type III). In all cases, an endoleak represents incomplete aneurysm exclusion with a risk of aneurysm rupture. Bernhard et al[24] have recently provided a detailed accounting of all reported cases of aneurysm rupture after endovascular repair, nearly all of which were related to endoleak. In a subgroup of 686 patients treated with Guidant/EVT endografts under FDA protocols, 5 instances of aneurysm rupture were identified. Hook fractures were contributory in most instances, and all events occurred in first-generation tube grafts. Two additional cases of rupture have been documented among a larger cohort of patients in whom Guidant/Ancure endografts were implanted after FDA market approval was granted on September 28, 1999. In both cases, the aneurysm was treated with a tube graft, albeit a second-generation device in which hook fracture was not a contributing factor. In an analysis of an additional 40 ruptures reported in the literature since 1995, most were caused by device failure, aneurysm remodeling, and inappropriate patient selection or device deployment, with an overall rupture-associated mortality rate of 50%. Ruptures occurred after implantation of a variety of endografts, including AneuRx, MinTec-Stentor (Mintec), Talent (World Medical, Sunrise, Fla), and Vanguard grafts, as well as other off-label devices. Although aneurysm rupture was most often associated with a type I or type III endoleak, this catastrophic event also occurred among patients who had no discernible endoleak or aneurysm expansion.

In the presence of a type I endoleak, options for endovascular salvage have included the reballooning of the attachment site and the placement of an additional cuff, extender, or stent. However, if the leak persists, open conversion is the most prudent course of action. Similarly, a type III endoleak caused by the disconnection of a modular prosthesis can, at times, be addressed by "tromboning" of additional graft components. Overall, 25% to 50% of type II endoleaks will seal spontaneously. However, some do persist and ruptures have been documented. Nonetheless, several groups have disputed that there is an inherent risk of rupture from type II endoleaks, and shrinking aneurysms with intrasac pressures that are substantially less than systemic values have been observed.[25]

Current estimates of the risk of aneurysm rupture after endovascular repair from an analysis of registry and multicenter trial data range from 0.6% to 2.6% per year.[26,27] Given the current state of the art, one can reasonably wonder whether overall rupture risk will ever be reduced to zero after endografting, even in the framework of a close surveillance program. As a corollary, a reduction of the risk for aneurysm rupture in the absence of complete protection may not provide sufficient compensation for the acknowledged limitations of open surgical repair in the younger patient at low risk for surgical intervention. A clear assessment of these issues will require continued careful analysis of the incidence and magnitude of the late complications of both open surgery and endovascular repair of aortic aneurysms. Certainly, further minimization of the risk of late device- or procedure-related complications will require additional improvements in device design and imaging technologies, as well as catheter-based procedures to salvage the failing endograft.

REFERENCES

1. Moore WS, Brewster DC, Bernhard VM: Aorto-uni-iliac endograft for complex aortoiliac aneurysms compared with tube/bifurcation en-dografts: Results of the EVT/Guidant trials. *J Vasc Surg* 33:S11-S20, 2001.
2. Zarins CK, White RA, Schwarten D, et al: AneuRx stent graft versus open surgical repair of abdominal aortic aneurysms: Multicenter prospective clinical trial. *J Vasc Surg* 29:292-305, 1999.
3. May J, White GH, Yu W, et al: Concurrent comparison of endoluminal versus open repair in the treatment of abdominal aortic aneurysms: Analysis of 303 patients by life table method. *J Vasc Surg* 27:213-220, 1998.
4. Berry AJ, Smith RB III, Weintraub WS, et al: Age versus comorbidities as risk factors for complications after elective abdominal aortic reconstructive surgery. *J Vasc Surg* 33:345-352, 2001.
5. Chaikof EL, Lin PH, Brinkman WT, et al: Endovascular repair of abdominal aortic aneurysms: Risk stratified outcomes. *Ann Surg* 235:833-841, 2002.
6. Henretta JP, Karch LA, Hodgson KJ, et al: Special iliac artery considerations during aneurysm endografting. *Am J Surg* 178:212-218, 1999.
7. Chuter TA, Reilly LM, Kerlan RK, et al: Endovascular repair of abdominal aortic aneurysm: Getting out of trouble. *Cardiovasc Surg* 6:232-239, 1998.
8. Armon MP, Wenham PW, Whitaker SC, et al: Common iliac artery aneurysms in patients with abdominal aortic aneurysms. *Eur J Vasc Endovasc Surg* 15:255-257, 1998.
9. Mehta M, Veith FJ, Ohki T, et al: Unilateral and bilateral hypogastric artery interruption during aortoiliac aneurysm repair in 154 patients: A relatively innocuous procedure. *J Vasc Surg* 33:S27-S32, 2001.
10. Lee WA, O'Dorisio J, Wolf YG, et al: Outcome after unilateral hypogastric artery occlusion during endovascular aneurysm repair. *J Vasc Surg* 33:921-926, 2001.
11. Holzenbein TJ, Kretschmer G, Thurnher S, et al: Midterm durability of abdominal aortic aneurysm endograft repair: A word of caution. *J Vasc Surg* 33:S46-S54, 2001.
12. Ohki T, Veith FJ, Shaw P, et al: Increasing incidence of midterm and long-term complications after endovascular graft repair of abdominal aortic aneurysms: A note of caution based on a 9-year experience. *Ann Surg* 234:323-335, 2001.
13. Schlensak C, Doenst T, Hauer M, et al: Serious complications that require surgical interventions after endoluminal stent-graft placement for the treatment of infrarenal aortic aneurysms. *J Vasc Surg* 34:198-203, 2001.
14. Bush RL, Lumsden AB, Dodson TF, et al: Mid-term results after endovascular repair of the abdominal aortic aneurysm. *J Vasc Surg* 33:S70-S76, 2001.

15. Daum RA, Shotty SK, Carpontor JP, et al: Limb kinking in supported and unsupported abdominal aortic stent-grafts. *J Vasc Interv Radiol* 11: 1165-1171, 2000.

16. Najibi S, Steinberg J, Katzen BT, et al: Detection of isolated hook fractures 36 months after implantation of the Ancure endograft: A cautionary note. *J Vasc Surg* 34:353-356, 2001.

17. Matsumura JS, Ryu RK, Ouriel K: Identification and implications of transgraft microleaks after endovascular repair of aortic aneurysms. *J Vasc Surg* 34:190-197, 2001.

18. Beebe HG, Cronenwett JL, Katzen BT, et al: Results of an aortic endograft trial: Impact of device failure beyond 12 months. *J Vasc Surg* 33:S55-S63, 2001.

19. Heintz C, Riepe G, Birken L, et al: Corroded nitinol wires in explanted aortic endografts: An important mechanism of failure? *J Endovasc Ther* 8:248-253, 2001.

20. Matsumura JS, Chaikof EL: Continued expansion of aortic necks after endovascular repair of abdominal aortic aneurysms. *J Vasc Surg* 28:422-430, 1998.

21. Prinssen M, Wever JJ, Mali WP, et al: Concerns for the durability of the proximal abdominal aortic aneurysm endograft fixation from a 2-year and 3-year longitudinal computed tomography angiography study. *J Vasc Surg* 33:S64-S69, 2001.

22. Cao P, Verzini F, Zannetti S, et al: Device migration after endoluminal abdominal aortic aneurysm repair: Analysis of 113 cases with a minimum follow-up period of 2 years. *J Vasc Surg* 35:229-235, 2002.

23. Conners MS, Sternbergh WC III, Carter G, et al: Endograft migration 1-3 years after endovascular AAA repair: A cautionary note. Transactions of the 26th Annual Meeting of the Southern Association for Vascular Surgery. Miami Beach, Fla, January 16-19, 2002.

24. Bernhard VM, Mitchell RS, Matsumura JS, et al: Ruptured abdominal aortic aneurysm following endovascular repair. *J Vasc Surg* 35:1155-1162, 2002.

25. Resch T, Ivancev K, Lindh M, et al: Persistent collateral perfusion of abdominal aortic aneurysm after endovascular repair does not lead to progressive change in aneurysm diameter. *J Vasc Surg* 28:242-249, 1998.

26. Harris PL, Vallabhaneni SR, Desgranges P, et al: Incidence and risk factors of late rupture, conversion, and death after endovascular repair of infrarenal aortic aneurysms: The EUROSTAR experience. *J Vasc Surg* 32:739-749, 2000.

27. Zarins CK, White RA, Moll FL, et al: The AneuRx stent graft: Four-year results and worldwide experience 2000. *J Vasc Surg* 33:S135-S145, 2001.

CHAPTER 9

Endovascular Management of Aortic and Iliac Aneurysms Using Multibranched and Fenestrated Stent-Grafts*†

Timothy A. M. Chuter, MD
Associate Professor of Surgery, Division of Vascular Surgery, University of California at San Francisco

A properly functioning stent-graft excludes the surrounding artery and all its branches from direct inflow. When the aneurysm itself has vital branches that cannot be deprived of flow, the stent-graft must also have branches. The simplest example is the use of a bifurcated stent-graft to treat an aneurysm at the aortic bifurcation. Each branch at the distal end of the stent-graft corresponds to a branch at the distal end of the aorta. This stent-graft configuration has become a familiar staple of endovascular surgery because the aneurysms are common. In addition, the insertion procedure is relatively simple because the common iliac arteries are large and easy to catheterize from downstream access points.

Branch artery encroachment is a more difficult problem in other locations, and it is fortunate that most abdominal aortic aneurysms end well below the renal arteries. The proximal and distal ends of the descending thoracic aorta are bounded by the subclavian and celiac arteries, whereas the proximal and distal ends of the aortoiliac segment are bounded by the renal and internal iliac arteries.

---

*Supported in part by grants from the Pacific Research Foundation.

†Dr Chuter has licensed patents to Cook Inc, manufacturer of the Zenith Device.

The renal and visceral arteries all arise from a short segment of aorta in between. Each location (aortic arch, visceral aorta, and common iliac bifurcation) requires its own distinct version of the multibranched approach.

GENERAL DESIGN CONSIDERATIONS

Multibranched and fenestrated stent-grafts share overlapping roles and, in some cases, overlapping technology. Both types of stent-graft are intended to exclude the aneurysm while maintaining flow to vital branches in the presence of compromised implantation sites. Fenestrated stent-grafts are useful when the branch artery arises close to the aneurysm; multibranched stent-grafts are needed when the branch artery arises from the aneurysm itself.

All the techniques of branch artery perfusion that have been explored to date represent points on the same continuum. At one end are the unibody stent-grafts of Inoue et al[1-3]; at the other are the fenestrated stent-grafts of Browne et al,[4-6] Park et al,[7] and Faruqi et al.[8] One has full-length branches, the other has only holes. Our grafts have short branches, which we extend into the branch arteries with additional components.[9] Another hybrid (Anderson) adds these extensions to a fenestrated graft, which otherwise would have only holes. In practical terms, the unibody approach[1-3] is distinct, requiring an ingenious system of catheters for deployment. The other techniques[4-9] share many similarities.

The short branches of our primary component enhance the seal between components and allow greater latitude for error in positioning at the expense of impaired sealing between the stent-graft and the aorta around the branch artery. With our device, this segment of the aorta has to be excluded from the circulation by moving the attachment site proximally to a supraceliac level. Fenestrated stent-grafts, on the other hand, seal to the margin of the branch artery and extend proximally only 1 to 2 cm above the aneurysm.

BILATERAL COMMON ILIAC ANEURYSMS

The usual way to deal with an iliac aneurysm is to occlude the internal iliac artery and implant the distal end of the stent-graft in the external iliac artery. Bilateral common iliac aneurysms present more of a problem, because bilateral internal iliac artery occlusion can cause intestinal ischemia, lumbosacral plexopathy, and severe buttock claudication.

There are several ways to maintain internal iliac perfusion under these circumstances, including external to internal iliac artery bypass, either by conventional surgical[10] or endovascular means.[11]

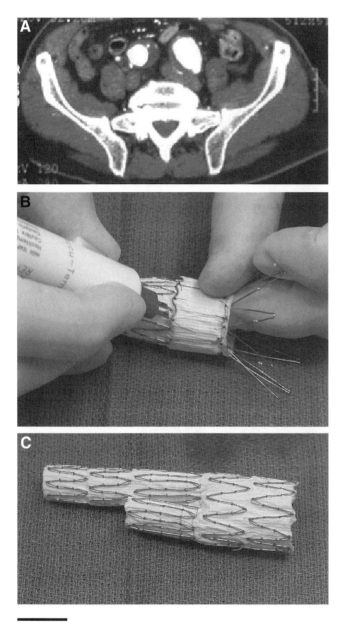

FIGURE 1.

A, Computed tomography showing bilateral common iliac aneurysms. B, Removal of the proximal half of a Zenith TFB-1-22 (Cook, Inc) main-body stent-graft using an ophthalmic cautery. C, The resulting bifurcated com-

(continued)

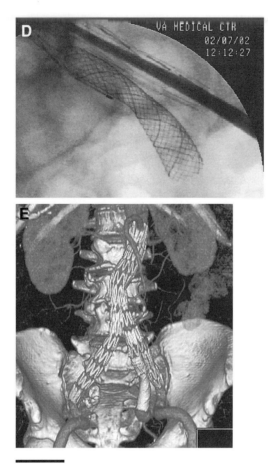

FIGURE 1. (continued)

mon iliac stent-graft. **D,** Fluoroscopy image of common iliac stent-graft implanted in the patient in **A.** The long leg is in the left external iliac artery, and there is a Wallgraft bridging the gap between the short leg and the internal iliac artery. **E,** Shaded surface rendering of the postoperative CT in the same patient, showing stent-graft bifurcations in the aorta and left common iliac artery.

We prefer to recreate the distal common iliac artery by using a bifurcated stent-graft (Fig 1). We make this bifurcated common iliac stent-graft from a small Zenith aortic stent-graft. The resulting prosthesis is implanted with the long leg in the external iliac artery and the body in the 20-mm-wide distal (common iliac) limb of a Zenith stent-graft. The short leg is extended into the internal iliac artery by inserting a 12-mm Wallgraft from a right brachial access point. We use 2 coaxial sheaths to reach the internal iliac artery from the right brachial artery: a 35-cm-long 14F sheath through the aortic arch, and an 80-cm-long 12F sheath through the stent-graft.

The first branched stent-grafts for iliac reconstruction were of the unibody type.[3] Other Zenith investigators have combined a modular system of aortic repair with a unibody bifurcated iliac component. Marin's system (originally Teramed, now Cordis) takes a similar approach.[12]

JUXTARENAL AORTIC ANEURYSMS

Browne et al[4-6] have developed a technique of stent-graft fenestration for juxtarenal aneurysms. The partially deployed Zenith main body stent-graft serves as a route of access to the renal artery (Fig 2). The bridging catheter is replaced over a wire for a small angioplasty balloon, which helps to guide the fenestration onto the renal orifice where it is fixed in position by a flared stent.

Although the principles remain the same, some technical details have changed in the years since it was first used. Current prac-

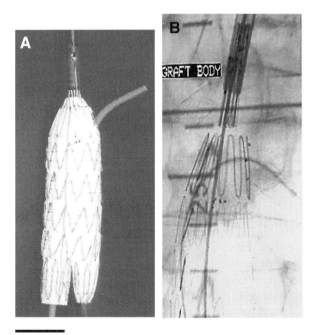

FIGURE 2.

A, Photograph of a fenestrated Zenith stent-graft. (Courtesy of M. Lawrence-Brown.) **B,** Intraoperative fluoroscopy showing a catheter traversing the stent-graft to the left renal artery.

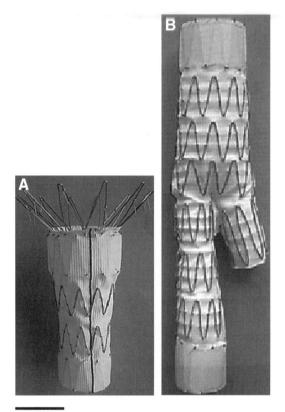

FIGURE 3.

A, Proximal fenestrated component of a Zenith composite main-body. **B,** Distal bifurcated component of a Zenith composite main-body.

tice is to separate the fenestrated proximal component from the bifurcated distal component (Fig 3). Once implanted, the 2 components of this "composite" main body share a long, wide, stable overlap. There are now 3 types of fenestration: a scallop, which is open proximally, a small fenestration, and a large fenestration. A stent-strut often crosses the orifice of the large fenestration, but not the scallop or small fenestration. The absence of a stent-strut facilitates the use of balloon-guided deployment and subsequent fixation with a bridging stent (Fig 4). When the stent-graft is properly oriented, the vertical line of anterior markers intersects the middle of the horizon-

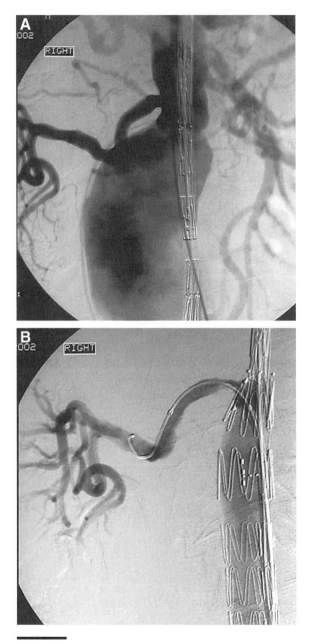

FIGURE 4.

A, Intraoperative angiogram showing the proximity of the right renal artery to the aneurysm. **B,** Intraoperative angiogram in the left anterior oblique view, showing a bridging wire extending from the main body through a scallop to the right renal

(continued)

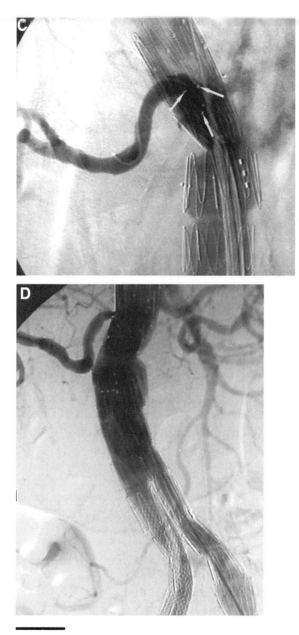

FIGURE 4. (continued)
artery. **C,** Intraoperative angiogram in the right anterior oblique view, showing the renal artery origin surrounded by radiopaque markers *(arrows)* on the edge of the scallop. **D,** Completion angiogram in the anteroposterior view, showing both components of the composite main-body Zenith stent-graft.

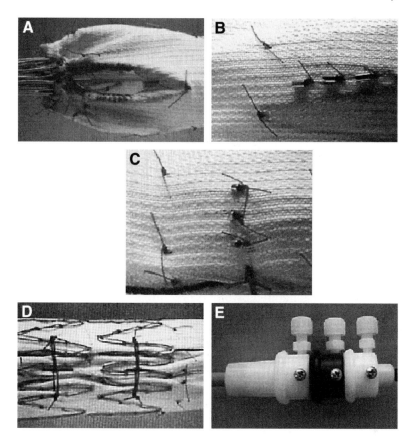

FIGURE 5.

A, A scallop in the space between 2 struts of the proximal sealing stent of a Zenith composite main body. **B,** A vertical line of radiopaque markers indicates the anterior aspect of the stent-graft. **C,** A horizontal line of markers indicates the posterior aspect of the stent-graft. **D,** The wall of the stent-graft is partially constrained by multiple suture loops around a trigger wire. **E,** Three trigger wires control deployment of the composite main-body stent-graft. The *outermost white ring* **(right)** controls graft expansion. The *black ring* controls proximal stent release. The *innermost white ring* **(left)** controls distal stent release.

tal line of posterior markers. The whole stent-graft is partially constrained by a series of loops around a trigger wire. In all, there are 3 trigger wires, controlling stent-graft expansion (white ring), proximal stent release (black ring), and distal stent-release (white ring), respectively, from the outer (distal) end inwards (Fig 5).

ANEURYSMS OF THE PROXIMAL DESCENDING THORACIC AORTA AND ARCH

Aneurysms of the proximal descending thoracic aorta and arch present several obstacles to endovascular repair. The aorta here is wide, compliant, and curved. The branches are clustered and feed an organ, the brain, with no tolerance for ischemia. A wide aorta requires a wide stent-graft. The delivery system is correspondingly bulky and stiff; often too wide to introduce through the iliac arteries and too stiff to introduce through the arch. Several stent-grafts have been developed for use in this location. Some have the required combination of flexibility, low profile, and trackability, but they are prone to late failure. These durability problems result in part from the compromises required for low profile, and in part from the cyclical stress and strain produced by the wide-ranging pulsatile movement of a compliant implantation site. Another late problem that tends to occur in this location is stent-graft migration. Marked aortic angulation impairs sealing and attachment, while increasing the displacement forces generated by blood pressure and flow.

Uncovered stents cannot be used to improve proximal attachment, because the curved aorta is susceptible to erosion and perforation by the tips of an uncovered stent. Moreover, an uncovered stent that crosses the left carotid or innominate artery origins could become a nidus for thrombus deposition and a source of ongoing embolism to the brain. The proximal end of the prosthesis has to have a covering of graft material, which limits its extension into the arch. Opinions vary as to the consequences of covering the subclavian artery, but clearly the graft cannot obstruct the left carotid artery without a high risk of stroke.

Fenestrated stent-grafts may have a role in this location because they enable the upstream end of the graft to move proximally into a more secure location without sacrificing flow to the branches of the distal arch. However, the necessary degree of accuracy in stent-graft orientation may be difficult to achieve. The self-orienting behavior of a preformed curve in the stent-graft or delivery system can help to establish the initial position, but resistance to rotation impedes subsequent attempts at fine-tuning. Once in place, the fenestration should probably be fixed in position by the addition of a bridging stent to minimize the risk of migration and subclavian or left carotid artery occlusion.

In theory, branched stent-grafts improve both fixation and sealing by embedding a side branch of the stent-graft in the subclavian artery. Single-branched, and even multibranched, stent-graft repair of the aortic arch appears feasible,[2] but reported complication rates have been high, and fundamental problems of stroke prevention, stent-graft delivery, and durability will have to be solved before this application has a major role.

In my opinion, the successful deployment of a multibranched unibody stent-graft is a feat of great skill, but not one that will ever be suitable for widespread application. The ingenious system used by Inoue et al[2] offers too many opportunities for error, all of which have dire consequences in this unforgiving location. The graft has multiple side branches, each with its own control catheter. Perhaps a modular approach would be simpler. Another possible simplification is the use of a single side branch, probably to the innominate artery. In this hybrid endovascular/open surgical technique, stent-graft implantation would be preceded by extra-anatomic bypass to the other brachiocephalic arteries.

ANEURYSMS OF THE DISTAL DESCENDING THORACIC AND THORACOABDOMINAL AORTA

Many of the problems encountered at the proximal end of the descending thoracic aorta are also found at the distal end. The segment of aorta between the aneurysm and the celiac artery is frequently short, conical, angulated, and ill-suited as an implantation site. Stent-graft fixation can be enhanced by adding an uncovered distal stent, but in many instances the graft itself must extend below the origin of the celiac to create a seal and prevent retrograde leakage into the aneurysm. When the aorta around the celiac artery is nondilated, anterior fenestration into the celiac and superior mesenteric arteries may suffice (Fig 6). When this area is actually part of the aneurysm, side branches are needed.

Our multibranched stent-graft[9] has 3 sets of components: a main body for the visceral aorta; tubular extensions for the renal, celiac, and superior mesenteric arteries; and a bifurcated system for the infrarenal aorta and common iliac arteries. The stent-graft attaches to the aorta above the aneurysm. Its branches are extended into the branches of the aorta by inserting small, flexible stent-grafts through a right brachial access. This technique has already been described in detail.[9]

The main body is a modified Zenith stent-graft with an uncovered proximal stent and 4 side arms (Fig 7). The diameter of the proximal end is sized to match the diameter of the supraceliac aorta,

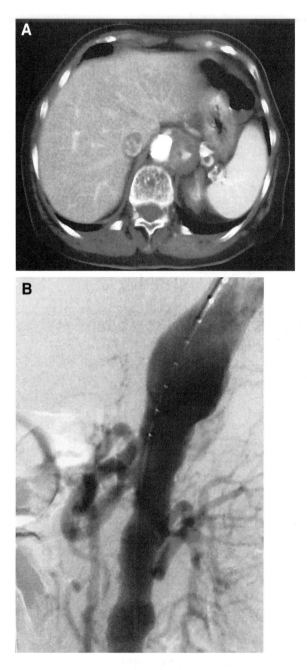

(continued)

but distally the graft narrows rapidly to allow space for all its branches. There are radiopaque markers at the proximal and distal ends of each branch. A second set of markers is used to establish and correct axial orientation. This component is delivered through a 20F or 22F sheath, depending on aortic diameter. The shaft of the delivery system carries 3 control wires just like those of the composite fenestrated stent-graft.

The visceral extensions were originally polytetrafluoroethylene-covered Smart stents (Cordis). We now use Hemobahn stent-

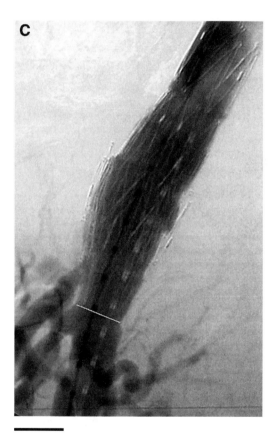

FIGURE 6. (continued)

A, Computed tomography showing contained rupture of a distal thoracic aortic aneurysm. **B,** Lateral angiogram in the same patient, showing a short conical segment of aorta between the aneurysm and the celiac artery. **C,** Completion angiogram (lateral view) showing the celiac artery, which is fed through a fenestration. The distal end of the stent-graft is indicated by the *white line.*

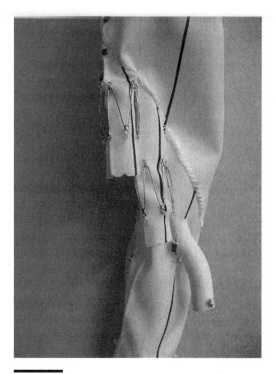

FIGURE 7.
The main body component of the thoracoabdominal stent-graft, showing side arms to the celiac, superior mesenteric, and left renal arteries. The other renal side arm is obscured.

grafts in 8- to 10-mm diameters and 5-cm lengths (Fig 8, A). We deliver these stent-grafts through a system of transbrachial sheaths very similar to (smaller diameter) the one used for bilateral iliac aneurysms. The infrarenal combination is essentially a Zenith TriFab system (Fig 8, B).

One problem with endovascular repair of thoraro abdominal aortic aneurysms (TAAAs) is the inability to reimplant intercostals arteries. We therefore avoid treating extensive type II and type III aneurysms (Fig 9) for fear of paraplegia. Other relative contraindications include multiple renal arteries; short renal arteries; stenoses of the renal, mesenteric, or celiac arteries; calcified, tortuous iliac arteries; and bilateral iliac aneurysms. The combination of iliac tortuosity and calcification impairs control of stent-graft orientation, and bilateral iliac aneurysms increase the risk of spinal ischemia. In addition, we would not perform endovascular repair of a TAAA in a

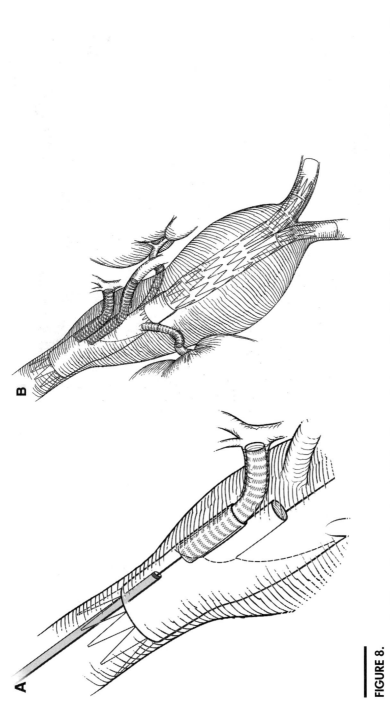

FIGURE 8.

A, Deployment of the celiac extension, bridging the gap between the celiac side arm of the main body and the celiac artery. **B,** When fully assembled, the thoracoabdominal stent-graft has 1 inflow and 5 branches.

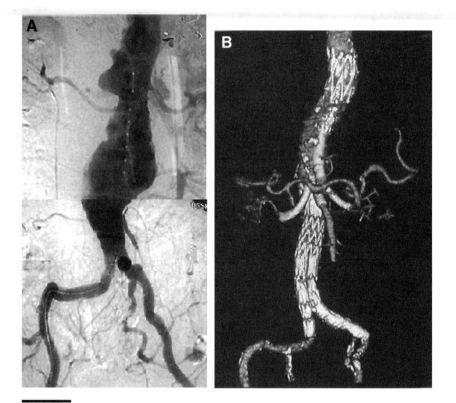

FIGURE 9.
A, Preoperative angiograms of a thoracoabdominal aortic aneurysm. In this case, there was a contained rupture of one of the proximal thoracic aortic ulcerations. **B,** Shaded surface rendering of postoperative computed tomography, after endovascular repair of this thoracoabdominal aneurysm.

patient fit for open repair. Given these restrictions, the population of suitable patients for the endovascular approach is very small.

PARARENAL ANEURYSMS

The combination of a Jomed stent-graft with a multifenestrated stent-graft has been used by John Anderson to treat a case of pararenal aneurysm. Because the fenestrated stent-graft has no branches, the resulting hybrid has no overlap zone between components, which may be something of a weak link. Historically, stent-grafts, such as the Stentor, with little or no overlap, have not been stable. Component separation led to type III endoleak and kinking.

We have developed a shortened version of our multibranched stent-graft for pararenal aneurysms (Fig 10) by minimizing the

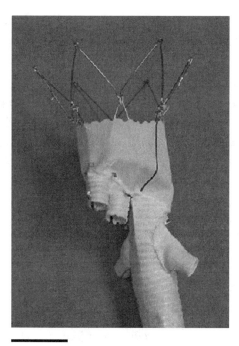

FIGURE 10.
The main body component of a stent-graft for pararenal aneurysms.

length of the supraceliac segment. The presence of side branches on this device precludes aortic implantation at or below the celiac artery. However, if these branches were shortened so as not to impinge on the surrounding aorta, the stent-graft could be placed over the visceral branches in the same manner as a fenestrated stent-graft, the difference being enhanced component-to-component attachment by virtue of the short cuffs.

CONCLUSION

Branched and fenestrated stent-grafts are no longer just a novelty. Participating centers in Australia and Europe have between them gained experience in more than 100 cases, with very good medium-term results. Of course, long-term results are needed before these techniques can be applied more widely. However, I believe that fenestrated and multibranched repairs are likely to be more durable than repairs that depend on the fate of a compromised proximal implantation site below the renal arteries. The aortic implantation site is the essential foundation of any endovascular repair, and these stent-grafts are able to take advantage of the healthiest segments of the aorta, while maintaining flow to branch arteries.

REFERENCES

1. Inoue K, Iwase T, Sato M, et al: Transluminal endovascular branched graft placement for a pseudoaneurysm: Reconstruction of the descending thoracic aorta including the celiac axis. *J Thorac Cardiovasc Surg* 114:859-861, 1997.
2. Inoue K, Hosokawa H, Iwase T, et al: Aortic arch reconstruction by transluminally placed endovascular branched stent graft. *Circulation* 100:SII316-SII321, 1999.
3. Iwase, T, Inoue K, Sato M, et al: Transluminal repair of an infrarenal aortoiliac aneurysm by a combination of bifurcated and branched stent grafts. *Cathet Cardiovasc Interv* 47:491-494, 1999.
4. Browne TF, Hartley D, Purchas S, et al: A fenestrated covered suprarenal aortic stent. *Eur J Vasc Endovasc Surg* 18:445-449, 1999.
5. Anderson JL, Berce M, Hartley DE: Endoluminal aortic grafting with renal and superior mesenteric artery incorporation by graft fenestration. *J Endovasc Ther* 8:3-15, 2001.
6. Stanley BM, Semmens JB, Lawrence-Brown MM, et al: Fenestration in endovascular grafts for aortic aneurysm repair: New horizons for preserving blood flow in branch vessels. *J Endovasc Ther* 8:16-24, 2001.
7. Park JH, Chung JW, Choo IW, et al: Fenestrated stent-grafts for preserving visceral arterial branches in the treatment of abdominal aortic aneurysms: Preliminary experience. *J Vasc Interv Radiol* 7:823, 1996.
8. Faruqi R, Chuter TAM, Reilly LM, et al: Endovascular repair of abdominal aortic aneurysm using a pararenal fenestrated stent-graft. *J Endovasc Surg* 6:354-358, 1999.
9. Chuter TAM, Gordon RL, Reilly LM, et al: An endovascular system for thoracoabdominal aortic aneurysm repair. *J Endovasc Ther* 8:25-33, 2001.
10. Parodi JC: Relocation of iliac artery bifurcation to facilitate endoluminal treatment of AAA. *J Endovasc Surg* 6:342-347, 1999.
11. Bergamini TM, Rachel ES, Kinney EV, et al: External iliac artery-to-internal iliac artery endograft: A novel approach to preserve pelvic inflow in aortoiliac stent grafting. *J Vasc Surg* 35:120-124, 2002.
12. Brener BJ, Faries P, Connelly T, et al: An in situ adjustable endovascular graft for the treatment of abdominal aortic aneurysms. *J Vasc Surg* 35:114-119, 2002.

CHAPTER 10

Advances in Imaging for Aortic Pathology

Mark F. Fillinger, MD

Associate Professor of Surgery, Section of Vascular Surgery, Dartmouth-Hitchcock Medical Center, Lebanon, NH

A dvances in imaging for surgical procedures tend to be directed pragmatically. In general surgery, the transition from open cholecystectomy to laparoscopic cholecystectomy produced a number of changes in intraoperative imaging, but few changes in preoperative imaging. Conversely, endovascular aortic aneurysm repair has required a radical change in preoperative planning, to insert a delivery system and place a permanently implanted device that requires precise tolerances for adequate "fit" and function of the device during the life of the patient. Thus, more precise, quantitative imaging methods have become mandatory for acute procedural success. Also, as the durability of endovascular repair comes into question, issues regarding proper patient selection, device selection, and postoperative surveillance become increasingly important for long-term success. These issues have driven changes in imaging for aortic pathology more than any other factor in recent years. Advances in "hardware" have also driven changes in imaging of vascular structures, but these tend to be less dramatic and more institution specific. For example, multidetector computed tomography (CT) scanners have decreased the imaging time while simultaneously improving collimation (beam thickness), allowing larger volumes to be imaged more quickly and without degradation in image quality. Although this is a great technical advance, it is largely transparent to the surgeon. In this update, recent "hardware" advances are covered briefly, but the focus is on how imaging is changing with regard to changes in surgical techniques.

HARDWARE

MAGNETIC RESONANCE ANGIOGRAPHY

Technological aspects of the equipment used for vascular imaging continue to improve rapidly. In the past, magnetic resonance angiography (MRA) has been limited by long acquisition times, resolution half that of CT, poor display of calcified plaque, and patient claustrophobia. Although these problems still exist with the standard equipment in most centers, most of them are being addressed with technology that will be more widely available in the future. Acquisition time in particular has limited the area and volume that can be imaged within a reasonable time frame, but the quality of studies with fast acquisition has greatly improved.[1,2] The continued development of blood-pool contrast media (eg, gadolinium) has improved the time window for acquisition, enhanced resolution of vascular structures, and improved the quality of 3-dimensional reconstruction from MRA.[3] Open configuration MR scanners are being developed for scanning during interventions (so-called open magnets). Although these are primarily used for neurosurgery and orthopedic

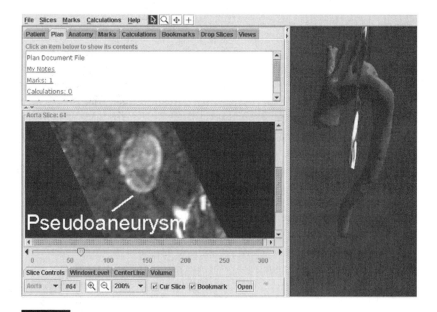

FIGURE 1.

MRA image with associated 3-dimensional reconstruction of a pseudoaneurysm of the thoracic aorta. The MRA reformat is displayed interactively within the 3-dimensional reconstruction to facilitate interpretation of the image.

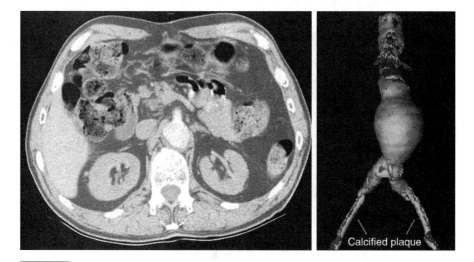

FIGURE 2.

CT scan with gadolinium contrast **(left)** and multiobject 3-dimensional reconstruction from the CT data. The 3-dimensional reconstruction is normally in 3 colors, but in this black-and-white reproduction, the thrombus/atheroma (yellow) and the calcified plaque (white) are both shades of gray. The contrast-enhanced lumen is in *dark gray*. The calcified plaque in this case is extensive **(right)** and would not be detected on MRA.

procedures at present, they may have vascular interventional uses in the future, and already show promise for diagnostic studies in patients with claustrophobia.[4-7] MRA is still very dependent on local protocols and postprocessing, much more so than CT, which is fairly standardized. Although the extremely high-quality MRA is still limited to 4 to 6 major centers of research, the quality of MRA at most medical centers is acceptable for 3-dimensional reconstruction (Fig 1). The problem of imaging calcified plaque remains a significant issue for vascular surgical procedures, and this is usually addressed by performing a noncontrast CT as an adjunctive study.[8] The other way to address cross-sectional diagnostic imaging for patients with renal insufficiency is to use gadolinium-enhanced CT (using typical "double-dose" or "triple-dose" for MRA, but diluted into 100 mL of normal saline for a typical CT volume infusion). Gadolinium does not provide the same density as iodinated contrast. Contrast enhancement is not as good as with iodinated contrast but is aided by adjusting the window level electronically on a CT workstation or equivalent. In general, gadolinium contrast is adequate for evaluation of the lumen and creation of a 3-dimensional reconstruction (Fig 2).

COMPUTED TOMOGRAPHY ANGIOGRAPHY

Spiral or helical CT is now standard in hospitals of almost any size. Software applications that recreate reformats of images in multiple planes (multiplanar reformats) and 3-dimensional reconstruction, which are often referred to generically as CT angiography (CTA), are also available on a basic level in most hospitals. Software continues to advance rapidly, and this will be addressed below. In terms of hardware, however, multidetector CT scanners are a significant advance and are already commonly available in major centers. One limit placed on standard single-row or single-detector spiral CT is emitter tube heat capacity, which limits the amount of time for the total scan, which in turn limits the beam thickness or collimation available when a long distance needs to be covered.[8] Increasing the beam thickness results in "averaging" of structures over the thickness of the "slice," which can lead to loss of resolution, averaging artifact, and failure to detect small branch vessels.[8] By using multiple detectors instead of the standard single row of detectors, a larger distance can be imaged with each rotation of the emitter without increasing the effective beam thickness. Thus, multidetector CT scanners can cover a longer distance along the "z" axis (from head to toe) in a shorter time without increasing the effective "thickness" of the slice that is imaged. For example, with 4-channel multidetector row CTA, vascular imaging over a distance of 1.2 mm (from the supraceliac abdominal aorta to the pedal arteries) can be imaged in 66 seconds, while still maintaining an effective section thickness of 3.2 mm.[9] Note that section thickness is not the same as reformat interval (the spacing between hard-copy prints, which can be set arbitrarily and is not a standard of quality—2-mm reformat interval with a section or beam thickness of 10 mm is useless). The "bottom line" is that multidetector row CT allows shorter acquisition times, greater coverage, and superior image resolution—basically superior to single-row scanners in every respect. Three-dimensional volume rendering is also improved, with capabilities for real-time, interactive modification of relative pixel attenuation in an infinite number of planes and projections. Already some investigators believe that this technique provides image quality that equals or surpasses that of conventional angiography.[10-12]

OPEN AORTIC ANEURYSM REPAIR

As described earlier, technological advances in hardware are substantial, but largely transparent to the surgeon. From a practical point of view the primary question is, how does this affect aortic imaging in routine practice? The answer to this question revolves primarily around the type of anatomic information that is required, which is often a function of the vascular procedure.

"SIMPLE" AORTIC ANEURYSM REPAIRS

Traditionally, imaging for the average abdominal aortic aneurysm (AAA) has not been extremely complex. Before high-quality CT, angiography was mandatory before open AAA repair, and later remained a frequently used adjunct.[13] As the capability to evaluate renal, mesenteric, and iliac artery occlusive disease improved during the past decade, however, diagnostic angiography is rarely required for repair of an infrarenal aorta.[14-17] A recent meta-analysis indicates that CTA or MRA with gadolinium contrast are the preferred studies for evaluation of potential renal artery stenosis.[18]

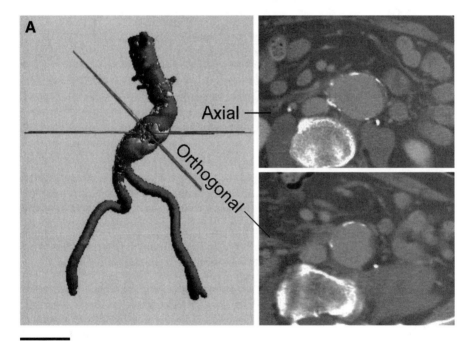

FIGURE 3.

A, Even mild AAA tortuosity can cause significant errors in diameter measurements by ultrasound. This patient was referred for an ultrasound measuring AAA diameter at 5 cm, when in reality the true maximum diameter was 4.1 cm using 3-dimensional reconstruction and appropriate orthogonal (perpendicular plane) reformats. The plane of ultrasound and the appropriate orthogonal plane are demonstrated within the context of the 3-dimensional reconstruction, but the ultrasonographer does not have this aid.

(continued)

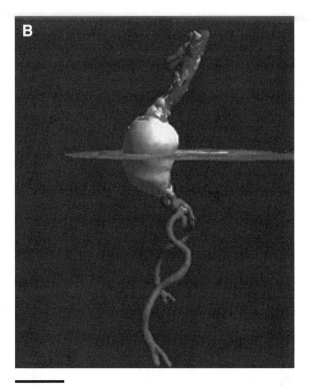

FIGURE 3. (continued)

B, This patient was referred for ultrasound AAA measurements of 5 to 5.5 cm, when in reality the true maximum diameter was 6.3 cm using 3-dimensional reconstruction and appropriate reformats. In this case, the ultrasound measurement missed the actual area of maximum diameter—again readily apparent on 3-dimensional reconstruction, but not apparent when scanning a patient through bowel gas and accompanying motion. The likely plane of ultrasound measurement is shown.

Some have suggested that ultrasound alone is sufficient for the typical, straightforward infrarenal AAA repair, but ultrasound and duplex ultrasound are very operator dependent and have pitfalls that may make the anatomic assessment misleading.[19] Even common problems such as mild tortuosity can cause significant errors in diameter measurements (Fig 3). It is important to remember that aortic aneurysm anatomy is usually a complex 3-dimensional structure, and even relatively sophisticated CT techniques can make aortic pathology appear more or less severe than it truly is (Fig 4). The other issue for apparently straightforward infrarenal AAAs is that most of these are now repaired by endovascular techniques at many centers.

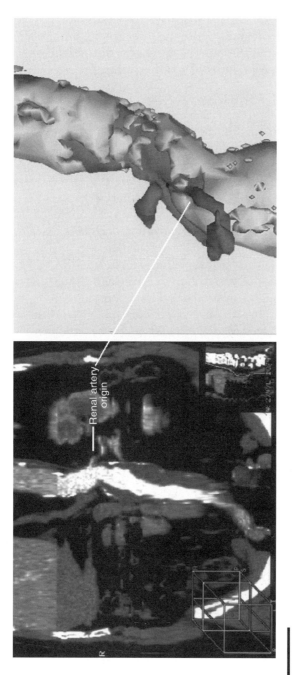

Renal artery origin

FIGURE 4.

Curvilinear reformat from spiral CT **(left)** displaying what appears to be a juxtarenal aortic aneurysm. Magnified view of multiobject 3-dimensional reconstruction **(right)** from the same CT demonstrates that the AAA is actually suprarenal. CT reformats do not always capture the key point of the anatomy, especially if they are not reproduced in sequential small intervals. Multiple visceral stenoses were also displayed on multiobject 3-dimensional reconstruction (not shown), including 2 that were missed on angiography but confirmed at the time of open surgery.

Most patients at least want a preliminary evaluation for potential endovascular repair, and realistically this requires CT. Of course, the remainder of aortic aneurysms—juxtarenal and suprarenal AAAs, thoracoabdominal or thoracic aortic aneurysms—clearly need to be evaluated with more sophisticated imaging.

COMPLEX AORTIC ANEURYSM REPAIRS

In the past, angiography was usually mandatory before the repair of complex aortic aneurysms, and this is still true in many centers. As spiral CT, multiplanar reformats, and 3-dimensional reconstruction have become available, however, the need for angiography has been minimized in many large centers. Several studies have demonstrated that even spiral CT with multiplanar reformats alone are accurate in delineating the extent of the aneurysm and evaluating significant renal, mesenteric, and iliac artery occlusive disease.[14-18,20] The need for angiography has been further lessened by the relatively widespread availability of gadolinium-enhanced MRA and multidetector scanners (as discussed above), as well as 3-dimensional reconstruction of CT and MRA with or without computer-aided measurement and planning software (as discussed in detail below). At Dartmouth-Hitchcock Medical Center, we rarely obtain angiography for open aortic surgery, but take care to use good CT scan protocols and optimal 3-dimensional reconstruction techniques.[8] We have found this method to be extremely reliable with regard to the extent of the aneurysm, branch vessel occlusive disease, and overall surgical planning.

THORACIC AORTA PATHOLOGY

Imaging of the thoracic aorta has always been associated with angiography, in part because of the difficulty of delineating dissections, traumatic aortic injury, and arch vessel occlusive disease. With the advent of fast scanners and spiral techniques, CT has become the study of choice in most of these cases.[8,21] Multidetector row scanners can cover the volume from the clavicles to the groins in 60 seconds and still maintain a relatively thin, effective slice thickness. Dissections remain difficult, but imaging techniques with 3-dimensional reconstruction of multiple objects (true lumen, false lumen, thrombus) have been found to be increasingly valuable (Fig 5).[21]

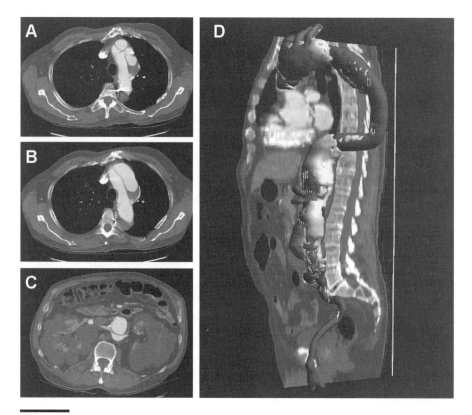

FIGURE 5.

Thoracoabdominal aortic dissection displayed on axial CT slices **(A-C)** and on 3-dimensional reconstruction with a sagittal slice inserted for improved context **(D)**. Determining continuity of the lumen can be difficult (note involvement of the innominate artery and relationship to the renal arteries on CT), but this can be greatly improved with multiobject CT. In this black-and-white reproduction, the red true lumen and magenta false lumen are unfortunately similar in gray. Atheroma and thrombus are *light gray* (normally yellow). Even in black and white, however, a very large amount of anatomic information is displayed rapidly with 3-dimensional reconstruction.

ENDOVASCULAR AORTIC ANEURYSM REPAIR

PREOPERATIVE IMAGING
CTA With Computer-Aided Measurement, Planning, and Simulation

Spiral CTA plus 3-dimensional reconstruction and specialized measurement software has emerged as an alternative to CT plus conventional angiography with a marker catheter. We have termed this more specialized technique "computer-aided measurement, planning, and simulation" (CAMPS), because the method incorporates more than simple CTA with 3-dimensional reconstructions. CAMPS includes the preferred elements of CTA with multiplanar reformats, CT reformats perpendicular (orthogonal) to the vessel, electronic measurements of highly magnified CT images, and spatially accurate 3-dimensional reconstructions (including multiobject reconstructions). Key diameter and length measurement problems are eliminated by combining these preferred techniques, and the cost and morbidity of an invasive test (angiography) are eliminated.[22-24] In cases of renal insufficiency, 3-dimensional reconstruction and multiplanar reformats can also be performed from MRA by using the same software, or from gadolinium-enhanced CT as described above.

CAMPS is probably best explained by a series of illustrations. Evaluation begins with CTA or MRA by using appropriate formatting (see above), including multiplanar reformats (sagittal, coronal,

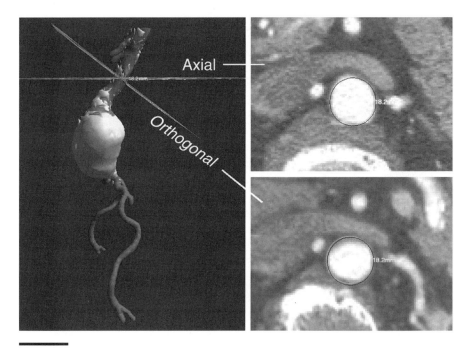

FIGURE 6.

Diameter measurements in the infrarenal aortic neck using axial or orthogonal reformats **(left)**. The *displayed marks* (reinforced in *black*) are identical in diameter, yet appear too small on the axial reformat **(upper right)** and appropriate (or perhaps even slightly large) on the orthogonal reformat **(lower right)**.

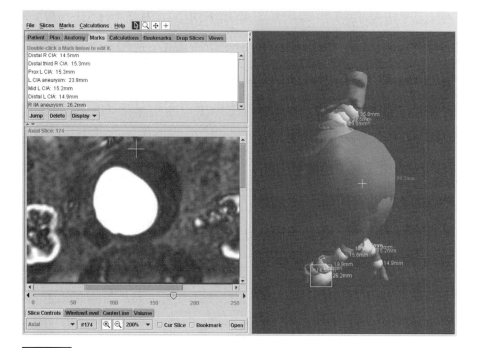

FIGURE 7.

MRA for a patient with renal insufficiency, and accompanying 3-dimensional reconstruction. The 3-dimensional display includes the set of diameter measurements typical for preoperative evaluation before endovascular AAA repair (external iliac measurements were also performed on CT without contrast). Note the appearance of thrombus on MR is a "void" rather than gray as on CT. Adjacent inferior vena cava, bowel, and spine also have a "void" appearance, so great care must be used for measurements and 3-dimensional reconstruction of elements outside the contrast-enhanced lumen on MRA. The *cross-hair* on the MRA slice corresponds to the *cross-hair* on the 3-dimensional reconstruction—all marks such as this are preferably displayed in both locations for better context.

and perpendicular to the vessel) throughout the entire area of interest. Multiobject 3-dimensional reconstructions are created based on the CT (or MR) density of the vessels,[8] and evaluated in an interactive way with the CT (or MR) data. The interactive evaluation clarifies some issues, such as the need for orthogonal reformats (perpendicular to the vessel) for accurate diameter measurements (Fig 6). Even in a subtle case such as this, the best possible measurements in magnified views with the use of electronic calipers result in a difference of 2 mm—a difference in selected stent-graft size for most manufacturers, or possibly the difference between an appropriate candidate and an inappropriate candidate for endovascular repair. It is also important to note that the error for diameter measurements on hard-copy films is twice that of measurements on an electronic workstation.[25] An appropriate evaluation includes the entire set of diameter and length measurements needed for endovascular repair, preferably in interactive fashion on an electronic workstation or equivalent (Fig 7). The preoperative CAMPS with 3-dimensional reconstruction is a very accurate representation of both the "angiogram view" and the completed endovascular repair, including the stent-graft configuration and end point simulated by the "virtual stent-graft" (Fig 8). In the illustrated case, preoperative CAMPS correctly predicted the appropriate diameters and lengths of the primary stent-graft and extension components for seal and fixation (which required an Ancure main device proximally and AneuRx extensions distally; no additional components were needed beyond those predicted preoperatively). We have found CAMPS evaluations and simulations to be extremely accurate, with no significant measurement errors in more than 200 endovascular AAA repairs without a preoperative angiogram (unpublished data). Moreover, we have found adjunctive angiography to be misleading in cases when CAMPS predicts difficult access.[22,26]

Creation of multiobject 3-dimensional reconstructions does have some disadvantages. This method is time-consuming even for experienced technicians. Physician time and training are required to provide an accurate and detailed analysis of hundreds of spiral CT reformat images and the 3-dimensional reconstruction itself. Nonetheless, this method can reveal anatomic abnormalities and potential problems for endovascular repair that may not be revealed by conventional spiral CT and angiography.[8,22-24,27] In many centers, CT plus 3-dimensional reconstruction and specialized measurement software is the method of choice because of equal or greater measurement accuracy than other methods, elimination of an invasive modality, and better patient selection.

FIGURE 8.

Computer-aided measurement, planning, and simulation (CAMPS) using MRA and its associated 3-dimensional model. **A,** Preoperative CAMPS/3-dimensional reconstruction with the thrombus made invisible to show only the contrast-enhanced lumen ("angiogram view"). Despite slight differences in magnification and viewing angle, this demonstrates an accurate representation of the anatomy displayed on
(continued)

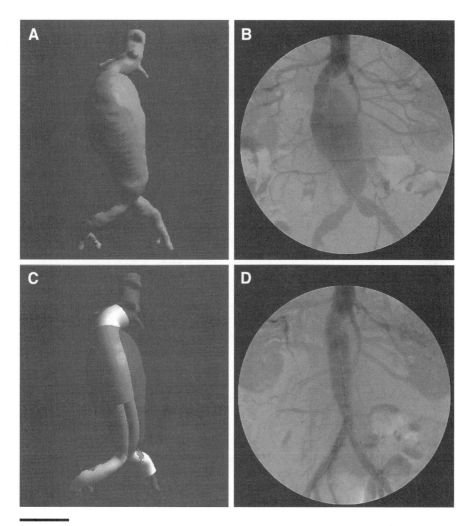

FIGURE 8. (continued)

the actual intraoperative angiogram **(B)**. **C,** The preoperative CAMPS/3-dimensional reconstruction is displayed with the thrombus invisible and blood flow transparent to better display the "virtual stent-graft" simulation. Despite slight differences in magnification, viewing angle, and straightening by guide wires, this preoperative simulation accurately predicts the stent-graft configuration and graft end points in the completed endovascular repair **(D)**. Note the indentation in the aortic neck (less apparent on virtual graft because the excess graft diameter is purposely displayed in the model), similar end point of the main trunk (Ancure endograft), the compression of the limbs at the aortic bifurcation, and the end points just proximal to the internal iliac arteries (taken before coil and cover of right internal iliac artery aneurysm not seen on angiogram).

Adjunctive Studies

Adjunctive studies regarding patient anatomy are generally not necessary after definitive anatomic characterization with CAMPS, but adjunctive studies with duplex, captopril renal scan, or MRA may sometimes be useful. A recent meta-analysis indicates that CTA or MRA with gadolinium contrast are the preferred studies for evaluation of potential renal artery stenosis,[18] and the evaluation must include an accurate evaluation of the superior mesenteric artery and inferior mesenteric artery, because the inferior mesenteric artery will be covered by the stent-graft. Therapeutic maneuvers for renal and iliac artery occlusive disease are generally avoided preoperatively. Renal stents often protrude into the aortic lumen and may complicate delivery and precise placement of the aortic stent-graft. Iliac angioplasty creates a dissection as part of the process, and this may cause "snow-plowing" of a large endovascular delivery device. Iliac stents can become terribly deformed and also complicate passage and delivery of these large delivery devices. Thus, iliac disease is treated by avoidance, bypass with iliac-femoral conduits, or the "Dotter" technique at the time of device delivery. Endovascular treatment of renal disease is generally avoided or treated after the aneurysm is excluded by the aortic stent-graft. As mentioned previously, evaluation of all these aspects can be accomplished well with CTA, CAMPS, or both.[8,14-18,20]

INTRAOPERATIVE IMAGING FOR ENDOVASCULAR INTERVENTIONS

A detailed description of specific endovascular AAA repair techniques is beyond the scope of this text, but some advances can affect the conduct of endovascular procedures. Traditionally, a preprocedure angiogram is obtained on the operating room table as a "road map" for delivery of the device. This is a time-tested portion of the procedure at this point, but it has some pitfalls. A large portion of AAAs have anteriorly angulated infrarenal "necks," which affect the appropriate angle of the c-arm gantry for optimal device deployment (Fig 9). Gantry angle simulation can also be performed for the internal iliac arteries. Knowing the location of the renal arteries in relation to the lumbar vertebrae (Fig 9) and the optimal gantry angle for the aortic neck and internal iliac arteries will avoid "trial and error" angiogram runs, excess dye load, and potential deployment errors with the device. For patients with severe renal insufficiency (but not on dialysis), we have used a combination of CAMPS, intravascular ultrasound (IVUS), and gadolinium or carbon dioxide (CO_2) to perform endovascular AAA repair without iodinated contrast. The density of the images with gadolinium and CO_2 is not as good as with

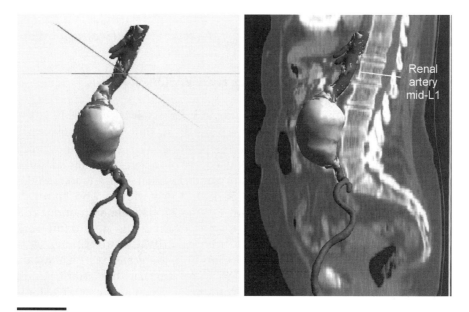

FIGURE 9.

Gantry angle simulation with planes cutting through the 3-dimensional model just below the lower renal artery **(left)**. This demonstrates how much of the infrarenal neck will be lost for fixation and sealing if the gantry is not adjusted to accommodate anterior angulation of the aorta in this location. In this patient, the loss of 5 to 10 mm of neck length will not be crucial, but a gantry angle error can be critical in patients with an available neck length of only 15 mm. On the **right** is a sagittal "drop slice" placed in a 3-dimensional model to determine the location of the lower renal artery relative to the lumbar vertebrae. This allows precise placement of the angiogram catheter at the time of the endovascular repair (avoiding contrast injections that fail to delineate the renal arteries or that heavily opacify overlying branches of the celiac and superior mesenteric artery).

iodinated contrast, so the use of IVUS and the road map of the preoperative 3-dimensional reconstruction are very helpful to the conduct of the procedure. The 3-dimensional reconstruction for these cases is obtained from MRA, CT without contrast, or CT with gadolinium because of the renal issues.[26] Caution should be used with CO_2 imaging, however, because of the risk of air emboli. CO_2 is also more difficult to use than gadolinium because it is less dense than blood and rises anteriorly, making viewing of the internal iliac arteries and renal arteries more difficult than with gadolinium. Gadolinium has dose restrictions, which limit its utility when angiogram information alone is used for an entire endovascular procedure. These restrictions make it almost mandatory to use 3-dimensional

Imaging, CAMPS, or IVUS to complement the available anatomic information and compensate for the relative deficits of gadolinium and CO_2.

POSTOPERATIVE IMAGING FOR ENDOVASCULAR AORTIC ANEURYSM REPAIRS

The long-term durability of endovascular repair is yet to be fully defined, so postoperative follow-up is crucial. Unfortunately, no single imaging modality is optimal for postoperative surveillance, so a combination of modalities is needed.[28] Current recommendations are for a clinic visit with history and physical examination, ankle-brachial indices, abdominal x-rays (3 or 4 views), and contrast-enhanced CT with or without 3-dimensional reconstruction. Abdominal x-rays are primarily used to evaluate the stent framework for deformation and fractures. CT is primarily used to evaluate stent-graft migration, fixation or apposition to the vessel wall, endoleak, branch vessels (renal, mesenteric, and internal iliac arteries), and aneurysm size (diameter and volume). CT can also evaluate stent-graft deformation and potential iliac occlusive disease in a manner that may supplement information obtained from ankle-brachial indices and abdominal x-rays. Duplex with color Doppler ultrasound or power Doppler can also be used to detect aneurysm size and potential endoleak, but accuracy tends to be on the order of 85%.[28,29] Contrast enhancement may increase accuracy, but duplex is highly operator dependent, subject to difficulties with bowel gas or obesity, and less accurate for determining migration and stent-vessel apposition. In addition, ultrasound is generally less accurate than CT for diameter measurements.[28,30]

The CT scanning protocol is crucial for postoperative evaluation of endografts. Contrast-enhanced CT should include the "arterial phase" at a minimum, with the addition of a noncontrast phase if extensive calcifications are present. Calcifications tend to "average" with low-density thrombus to produce an intermediate density that can be confused with contrast enhancement.[28] A noncontrast CT can be performed with thicker collimation to prevent x-ray emitter tube overheating before the arterial phase CT, although this is becoming less problematic with newer CT hardware. If the aneurysm enlarges at any time point, or shows no signs of shrinkage within 1 year, evaluation should be directed toward finding a potential endoleak or attachment site problem. If there is no evidence of endoleak on arterial phase CT, a "venous phase" CT should be performed. The venous phase spiral can be performed with a 2- to 5-minute delay after the arterial phase, again using thicker collimation to avoid tube overheating if necessary. The venous phase technique can detect smaller, late-filling endoleaks that are not easily detected by other means.[28,31] If no endoleak is detected with the delayed venous phase technique, consideration should be given to transmission of pressure without actual flow of contrast or "endotension."[32] Pressure transmission can occur through thrombus when the stent-graft is seated in thrombus rather than seated against the vessel adventitia, or when a small hole is sealed with thrombus.[31,33] Three-dimensional reconstruction of CT or MRA data (including special reformats and magnified views) can be extremely useful for detecting the source of an endoleak, for evaluating appropriate fixation, and for detecting shape and volume changes. Our group and others have demonstrated that aneurysm enlargement is more accurately detected by volume changes than by diameter changes.[28,34] In a recent multicenter analysis of adverse events after endovascular AAA repair, the only postoperative parameter that predicted the majority of ruptures was AAA volume change, and in several cases, volume change demonstrated a problem 12 months before rupture occurred.

Follow-up is currently recommended at 1 month, 6 months, and 12 months postoperatively. Thereafter, follow-up should be at 6- or 12-month intervals. More frequent follow-up or intervention is generally required when endoleak is detected or when the aneurysm is not clearly shrinking. Currently, repair is recommended for all type I (attachment site) endoleaks, type III (graft material defects or modular junction separation) endoleaks, and any endoleak with signs of aneurysm expansion. At present, isolated type II endoleaks (with no associated type I or III endoleaks) appear to be more benign than other types of endoleak, and intervention is only necessary when the AAA is enlarging by volume or diameter.[35] Intervention will also be necessary for cases of stent-graft deformation that lead to occlusions. Correction for endoleak and occlusion may be via endovascular or open repair, but in most cases endovascular repair is possible.[36] At present, annual follow-up with imaging studies should be considered mandatory for the life of the patient, since a number of problems occur more than 1 year after endovascular AAA repair,[36] and the frequency of problems continues to be significant thereafter.[35,37]

REFERENCES

1. Ruehm SG, Goyen M, Barkhausen J, et al: Rapid magnetic resonance angiography for detection of atherosclerosis. *Lancet* 357:1086-1091, 2001.

2. Pereles FS, McCarthy RM, Baskaran V, et al. Thoracic aortic dissection and aneurysm: Evaluation with nonenhanced true FISP MR angiography in less than 4 minutes. *Radiology* 223:270-274, 2002.

3. Vosshenrich R, Fischer U: Contrast-enhanced MR angiography of abdominal vessels: Is there still a role for angiography? *Eur Radiol* 12:218-230, 2002.

4. Lipson AC, Gargollo PC, Black PM: Intraoperative magnetic resonance imaging: Considerations for the operating room of the future. *J Clin Neurosci* 8:305-310, 2001.

5. Woodard EJ, Leon SP, Moriarty TM, et al: Initial experience with intraoperative magnetic resonance imaging in spine surgery. *Spine* 26:410-417, 2001.

6. Bohinski RJ, Warnick RE, Gaskill-Shipley MF, et al: Intraoperative magnetic resonance imaging to determine the extent of resection of pituitary macroadenomas during transsphenoidal microsurgery. *Neurosurgery* 49:1133-1143, 2001.

7. Spouse E, Gedroyc WM: MRI of the claustrophobic patient: Interventionally configured magnets. *Br J Radiol* 73:146-151, 2000.

8. Fillinger MF: Computed tomography, CT angiography and three-dimensional reconstruction for the evaluation of vascular disease, in Rutherford RB (ed): *Rutherford's Textbook of Vascular Surgery*, ed 5. Philadelphia, WB Saunders, 2000, pp 230-268.

9. Rubin GD, Schmidt AJ, Logan LJ, et al: Multi-detector row CT angiography of lower extremity arterial inflow and runoff: Initial experience. *Radiology* 221:146-158, 2001.

10. Macari M, Israel GM, Berman P, et al: Infrarenal abdominal aortic aneurysms at multi-detector row CT angiography: Intravascular enhancement without a timing acquisition. *Radiology* 220:519-523, 2001.

11. Roos JE, Willmann JK, Weishaupt D, et al: Thoracic aorta: Motion artifact reduction with retrospective and prospective electrocardiography-assisted multi-detector row CT. *Radiology* 222:271-277, 2002.

12. Lawler LP, Fishman EK: Multi-detector row CT of thoracic disease with emphasis on 3D volume rendering and CT angiography. *Radiographics* 21:1257-1273, 2001.

13. Brewster DC, Retana A, Waltman AC, et al: Angiography in the management of aneurysms of the abdominal aorta: Its value and safety. *N Engl J Med* 292:822-825, 1975.

14. Galanski M, Prokop M, Chavan A, et al: Renal arterial stenoses: Spiral CT angiography. *Radiology* 189:185-192, 1993.

15. Cikrit DF, Harris VJ, Hemmer CG, et al: Comparison of spiral CT scan and arteriography for evaluation of renal and visceral arteries. *Ann Vasc Surg* 10:109-116, 1996.

16. Raptopoulos V, Rosen MP, Kent KC, et al: Sequential helical CT angiography of aortoiliac disease. *Am J Roentgenol* 166:1347-1354, 1996.

17. Kaatee R, Beek FJ, Verschuyl EJ, et al: Atherosclerotic renal artery stenosis: Ostial or truncal? *Radiology* 199:637-640, 1996.

18. Vasbinder GB, Nelemans PJ, Kessels AG, et al: Diagnostic tests for renal artery stenosis in patients suspected of having renovascular hypertension: A meta-analysis. *Ann Intern Med* 135:401-411, 2001.

19. Nguyen D, Hamper UM: False positive dissection of abdominal aortic aneurysm by color Doppler duplex ultrasonography. *J Ultrasound Med* 14:467-469, 1995.

20. Van Hoe L, Baert AL, Gryspeerdt S, et al: Supra- and juxtarenal aneurysms of the abdominal aorta: Preoperative assessment with thin-section spiral CT. *Radiology* 198:443-448, 1996.

21. Fillinger MF: Imaging of the thoracic and thoracoabdominal aorta. *Semin Vasc Surg* 13:247-263, 2000.

22. Fillinger MF: New imaging techniques in endovascular surgery. *Surg Clin North Am* 79:451-475, 1999.

23. Broeders I, Blankensteijn J, Olree M, et al: Preoperative sizing of grafts for transfemoral endovascular aneurysm managment: A prospective comparative study of spiral CT angiography, arteriography, and conventional CT imaging. *J Endovasc Surg* 4:252-261, 1997.

24. Beebe HG, Jackson T, Pigott JP: Aortic aneurysm morphology for planning endovascular aortic grafts: Limitations of conventional imaging methods. *J Endovasc Surg* 2:139-149, 1995.

25. Aarts NJ, Schurink GW, Schultze Kool LJ, et al: Abdominal aortic aneurysm measurements for endovascular repair: Intra- and interobserver variability of CT measurements. *Eur J Vasc Endovasc Surg* 18:475-480, 1999.

26. Fillinger MF, Weaver JB: Imaging equipment and techniques for optimal intraoperative imaging during endovascular interventions. *Semin Vasc Surg* 12:315-326, 1999.

27. Fillinger MF: Utility of spiral CT in the preoperative evaluation of patients with abdominal aortic aneurysms, in Whittemore AD (ed): *Advances In Vascular Surgery*, vol 5. St Louis, Mosby, 1997, pp 115-131.

28. Fillinger MF: Postoperative imaging after endovascular AAA repair. *Semin Vasc Surg* 12:327-338, 1999.

29. Sato DT, Goff CD, Gregory RT, et al: Endoleak after aortic stent graft repair: Diagnosis by color duplex ultrasound scan versus computed tomography scan. *J Vasc Surg* 28:657-663, 1998.

30. Thomas PR, Shaw JC, Ashton HA, et al: Accuracy of ultrasound in a screening programme for abdominal aortic aneurysms. *J Med Screen* 1:3-6, 1994.

31. Schurink GW, Aarts NJ, Wilde J, et al: Endoleakage after stent-graft treatment of abdominal aneurysm: Implications on pressure and imaging: An in vitro study. *J Vasc Surg* 28:234-241, 1998.

32. Gilling-Smith GL, Martin J, Sudhindran S, et al: Freedom from endoleak after endovascular aneurysm repair does not equal treatment success. *Eur J Vasc Endovasc Surg* 19:421-425, 2000.

33. Marty B, Sanchez LA, Ohki T, et al: Endoleak after endovascular graft repair of experimental aortic aneurysms: Does coil embolization with

anglographic "seal" lower intraaneurysmal pressure? *J Vasc Surg* 27. 454-461, 1998.

34. Balm R, Kaatee R, Blankensteijn JD, et al: CT-angiography of abdominal aortic aneurysms after transfemoral endovascular aneurysm management. *Eur J Vasc Endovasc Surg* 12:182-188, 1996.

35. Marrewijk C, Buth J, Harris PL, et al: Significance of endoleaks after endovascular repair of abdominal aortic aneurysms: The EUROSTAR experience. *J Vasc Surg* 35:461-473, 2002.

36. Umscheid T, Stelter WJ: Time-related alterations in shape, position, and structure of self-expanding, modular aortic stent-grafts: A 4-year single-center follow-up. *J Endovasc Surg* 6:17-32, 1999.

37. Laheij RJ, Buth J, Harris PL, et al: Need for secondary interventions after endovascular repair of abdominal aortic aneurysms: Intermediate-term follow-up results of a European collaborative registry (EUROSTAR). *Br J Surg* 87:1666-1673, 2000.

C HAPTER 11

Laparoscopic Vascular Surgery: Perspectives

Yves-Marie Dion, MD, MSc
Professor, Department of Surgery, Laval University and Centre
Hospitalier Universitaire de Québec, Hôpital Saint-François d'Assise,
Québec, Canada

Yvan Douville, MD, MSc
Professor, Department of Surgery, Laval University and Centre
Hospitalier Universitaire de Québec, Hôpital Saint-François d'Assise,
Québec, Canada

Carlos R. Gracia, MD
Associate Professor, Department of Surgery, University of California, Los
Angeles

Fabien Thaveau, MD
Fellow, Department of Surgery, Centre Hospitalier Universitaire de
Québec, Hôpital Saint-François d'Assise, Québec, Canada

In the early 1990s, laparoscopic treatment of aortoiliac aneurysmal or occlusive disease was unheard of. However, numerous laparoscopic techniques had been developed to perform cholecystectomy, antireflux procedures, colon resection, splenectomy, adrenalectomy, and others. In this chapter, we describe the history that led to the performance of the first assisted aortobifemoral (ABF) bypass and to the first totally laparoscopic ABF bypass. We present the results of our laparoscopic work in the field of occlusive and aneurysmal disease. We also review advances in technology that occurred during that time and had an impact on our work and that of others.

After the excellent results of laparoscopic techniques in general surgery, we attempted in 1991 to develop a laparoscopic treatment for aortoiliac disease. Our initial goals were to reduce mortality, morbidity, postoperative pain, and hospital stay while providing the patient with the excellent patency rates attributed to standard bypass surgery.

Advances in Vascular Surgery®, vol 10

HISTORY OF LAPAROSCOPIC VASCULAR ACCESS: DEVELOPMENT OF A NEW CONCEPT

LABORATORY EXPERIMENTS: LAPAROSCOPY-ASSISTED TECHNIQUE

Approach: Gasless Versus Pneumoperitoneum

In 1991, our early laboratory work to evaluate a possible access and exposure of the aorta was done by using an original abdominal wall lifting device (Laborie Surgical, Ltd, Longueuil, Quebec). Prototype clamps and forceps were also designed by the same company. We later used the Laparolift, designed by Origin MedSystems, Menlo Park, California. We thought that a gasless approach with an abdominal lift device would serve 2 purposes: avoid potential air embolisms associated with pneumoretroperitoneum in the event of a venous injury, and maintain open the retroperitoneal space even if heavy suctioning was needed.

However, we later demonstrated that the risk of significant air embolism was very low and that loss of pneumoperitoneum was not an important issue.[1] In this experiment, dogs had hemodynamic monitoring via an arterial line and Swan-Ganz catheter. Transesophageal echocardiography was used to evaluate the status and amount of embolism within the heart chambers. Under carbon dioxide (CO_2) pneumoperitoneum, euvolemic dogs were submitted to a 1-cm longitudinal incision made into the inferior vena cava while maintaining a CO_2 pneumoperitoneum with pressures varying between 12 and 15 mm Hg. No gas embolism was seen in 82% of the cases after exposure of the venotomies to the pneumoperitoneum (Fig 1, A and B). Only 18% had some gas bubbles visible in the right heart cavities by transesophageal echocardiography. In contrast, direct intravenous bolus injection in the internal jugular vein of only 15 mL of CO_2 led to visualization of many more gas bubbles in the right heart cavities (Fig 1, C and D). Massive intravenous injections of CO_2 (>300 mL) led to the appearance of gas bubbles in the left heart cavities and death (Fig 1, E). After this experiment, we concluded that CO_2 insufflation could be used safely in laparoscopic vascular surgery.

Another advantage of using CO_2 insufflation was that it could be used to gain access to the aorta by helping in the dissection and distention of the retroperitoneum. We attempted other techniques such as hydrodissection and balloon dissection of the retroperitoneum. We found that the former technique left edematous tissues, whereas the latter could be a useful adjunct to the procedure with some tech-

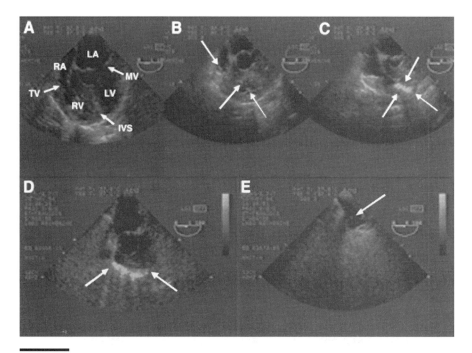

FIGURE 1.

A, Normal canine heart. The open tricuspid valve *(TV)* separates the right atrium *(RA)* from the right ventricle *(RV)*. The interventricular septum *(IVS)*, the left ventricle *(LV)*, the left atrium *(LA)*, and the mitral valve *(MV)* are seen. **B,** A few CO_2 bubbles are visualized in the RA and RV *(arrows)* after caval venotomy. **C,** More gas bubbles are seen in the RV after injection of 15 mL into the jugular vein *(arrows)*. **D,** Injection of 100 mL of CO_2 leads to a larger gas embolus *(arrows)*, which led to a significant increase in the pulmonary artery pressure. **E,** Massive air embolism after injection of 300 mL of CO_2, leading to the death of the animal. The RA, RV, and LV, are totally obscured by embolism material, and gas bubbles *(arrow)* are visible in the LA.

nical modifications. We settled on dissection done with the laparoscope under CO_2 insufflation.

Development of Laparoscopic Transabdominal Retroperitoneal Approach

Our first successful animal work[2] consisted of performing a patch aortotomy in dogs (Fig 2, A and B). At the time, laparoscopic exposure of the aorta was not possible. Before the laparoscopic aortotomy, therefore, laparotomy was undertaken for placement of retractors and ligation of lumbar arteries after transperitoneal incision of the retroperitoneum. We rapidly recognized that to obtain a clear view of the retroperitoneal structures, time-consuming and tedious laparoscopic retraction of the intraperitoneal organs was mandatory. Moreover, the transperitoneal approach required suturing the retroperitoneum over the prosthesis at the end of the procedure, a difficult technical exercise in itself. Consequently, we devised a retroperitoneal technique that not only would facilitate exposure but would also reduce the risk of iatrogenic injury to the bowel.

During the same period, we performed the first human laparoscopy-assisted ABF bypass[3] (Fig 3, A). In our mind, this technique, which requires a limited laparotomy, was the first step toward the development of the totally laparoscopic technique under investigation in the laboratory. Six patients underwent laparoscopy-assisted ABF bypass (Fig 3, B and C). The last 3 were submitted to what is now called hand-assisted laparoscopic surgery (Fig 3, D-F). All patients demonstrated improved postoperative courses characterized by early ambulation with less pain and less need for analgesics. One patient sustained a small bowel perforation from difficult retraction, a potential source of injury inherent in the transperitoneal approach. Operative details include the use of pneumoperitoneum, dissection of the aortoiliac segment, and tunneling of the graft, all completed laparoscopically. Then a small minilaparotomy was performed to construct an end-to-side aortic anastomosis.

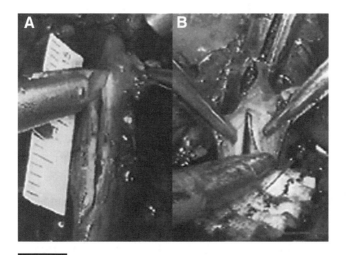

FIGURE 2.
Our first successful laparoscopic aortic patch. **A,** Creation of the aortotomy. **B,** The needle has been passed through the Dacron patch, and its tip is penetrating the arterial wall.

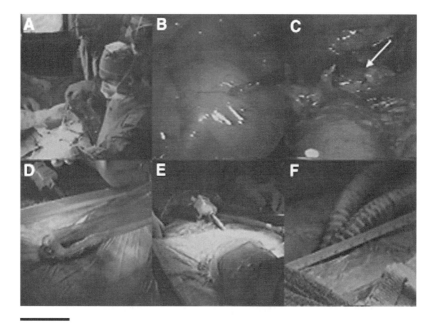

FIGURE 3.
A, First human laparoscopy-assisted aortobifemoral bypass. B and C, Laparoscopy-assisted procedure (transperitoneal approach, 1993) demonstrating a forceps at the aortic bifurcation (**B**) and the left renal vein (**C,** *arrow*). D and E, First hand-assisted procedure (transperitoneal approach, 1993) for treatment of aortoiliac disease. F, Proximal anastomosis has been done through a 6- to 8-cm skin incision.

We noticed some potential limitations of the laparoscopy-assisted approach. With increasing thickness of the abdominal wall, the incision must be lengthened to achieve good exposure, thereby negating the potential advantage sought by minimizing surgical trauma. This clinical experience also confirmed the difficulty associated with the transperitoneal route with respect to bowel retraction. Available laparoscopic instrumentation failed to provide expeditious retraction of intra-abdominal organs, and aortic dissection and proximal aortoprosthetic anastomosis proved extremely tedious. The retroperitoneal approach appeared to be the solution, since the retroperitoneum could function as an organ retractor and also provide excellent exposure of the major vessels.

In the laboratory, piglets were selected because their retroperitoneal anatomy is comparable to human beings, despite their smaller caliber arteries. The Yorkshire-cross piglet weighs 75 to 80

kg and approximates working in the human torso, yet the aorta typically measures 10 to 11 mm in diameter. However, when clamped
and transected, the aorta contracts, so a 6-mm graft is an appropriate
match for anastomosis. This finding required a 6 mm/6 mm aortic
prosthesis constructed from grafts 6 mm in diameter and sewn to
each other in an end-to-side fashion to form an appropriate bifurcated prosthesis. However, based on our clinical experience to date,
the larger human aorta (a 14- or 16- mm-diameter prosthesis being
used) has proven technically easier to work with because its size
facilitates many of the maneuvers used in laparoscopic suturing,
such as handling of the needle during the anastomosis. The second
limitation is that the porcine vessels have no atherosclerosis. Successful animal work would not ensure that available instrumentation and laparoscopic suture techniques would prove applicable in
the presence of plaque. As clinical experience evolved, we found
that atheromatous plaque could be handled laparoscopically in a
manner similar to open cases. Laparoscopic tools provided tactile
feedback comparable to conventional open instrumentation feedback so essential to a surgeon working with instruments.

Our group reported the first laparoscopic experience consistently with the use of a retroperitoneal approach.[2] The anterior laparoscopic approach described by Schumacker was initially attempted, but abandoned in favor of the lateral approach to access
the retroperitoneum. With the piglets in the right lateral decubitus
position, retroperitoneal dissection (aided by balloon dissectors)
created the retroperitoneal space. The aorta was visualized and dissected from the left renal artery to the bifurcation. Abdominal wall
suspension was used, and total laparoscopic aortoprosthetic anastomoses were performed. Exposure of the femoral vessels, and subsequent tunneling of the prosthetic graft to the groins, required the
animal to be turned to a more supine position for completion of the
bypass.

Despite this successful experience, it became apparent that to
completely translate this approach to actual human application, it
would be necessary to modify the patient's position on the operative
table. We then designed in the laboratory an anterolateral laparoscopic approach for human laparoscopic ABF bypass.[4] This approach allowed the surgeon and an assistant to work in the same
fashion as if the abdomen was opened. The procedure was originally described in which a gasless technique was used. The goal was
not only to reproduce the exposure and control achieved by the lateral approach, but to more completely expose and control the distal
aorta and iliac arteries. Exposure and control of the inferior mesen-

teric artery and lumbar vessels were also necessary. Uncontrolled lumbar vessels at the time of incision or division of the aorta could result in sufficient bleeding to obscure the operative laparoscopic view. Although total laparoscopic ABF bypass was being safely carried out, difficulties inherent to the gasless technique led to the performance of the procedure under pneumoperitoneum.

After further animal studies and cadaver work, we developed a modified technique in which the peritoneum was used as a protective shield against intrusion of intraperitoneal organs in the working field.[5] The "apron technique" also eliminates the threat of competitive insufflation favoring one cavity versus the other (intraperitoneal vs extraperitoneal) since both cavities are interconnected.

To evaluate the possibility of developing a totally laparoscopic approach to aortic aneurysmal repair, a method was designed whereby the aorta was opened longitudinally after proximal and distal control. The lumbar arteries were controlled not only from outside the aorta, but also oversewn while bleeding from within the lumen as in open repair. The anastomosis was constructed in an end-to-end fashion by suturing from within the aorta and incorporating an intact posterior wall to reproduce the conventional open technique. All anastomoses were constructed with continuous standard monofilament 4-0 Prolene suture on curved vascular needles. Construction of the ABF bypass was consistently achieved in less than 4 hours.[6] All anastomoses were patent without stenoses with the graft limbs correctly tunneled under the ureters. Blood loss never exceeded 550 mL, most of which occurred at the time the aorta was opened and flushed. On occasion, bleeding appeared from the oversewn aortoiliac stump after the limbs of the grafts were opened, and additional sutures were applied as necessary. In these early models, the totally laparoscopic aortic anastomosis did not take more than 60 minutes to perform. The magnification afforded by a well-placed laparoscope allowed an excellent view for meticulous completion of the anastomosis. No operative mortality was encountered in piglets, which together accounted for 34 consecutive totally laparoscopic ABF bypasses.[2,4,6]

THE FIRST HUMAN TOTALLY LAPAROSCOPIC PROCEDURE: THE CLINICAL PROTOCOL

Originally, patients enrolled for ABF bypass were treated according to a research protocol accepted by le Centre Hospitalier Universitaire de Québec, Pavillon St-François d'Assise ethics committee. The main inclusion criteria of the protocol were symptomatic aortoiliac occlusive disease that could not be treated by percutaneous

TABLE 1.
Exclusion Criteria

Aortoiliac disease that could be treated by percutaneous
  transluminal angioplasty
Prior left hemicolectomy
Thrombosis of the aorta up to the renal arteries
Horseshoe kidney or polar arteries
Unfit for surgery
Morbid obesity (weight greater than 100% ideal weight)
Cardiac or pulmonary contraindications to laparoscopy
Renal insufficiency
Juxtarenal aneurysm
Large aortobiiliac aneurysm
Psychiatric disease

transluminal angioplasty. Only patients able to sign an informed consent form could be included in the trial. Current exclusion criteria are listed in Table 1. A preoperative computed tomography scan is done to identify anatomic variation of the intra-abdominal veins (retroaortic left renal vein, double inferior cava) or organs (horseshoe kidneys), and to detect significant calcification of the aorta. A preoperative angiogram should define the renal (inferior polar renal artery) and visceral vascular anatomy. Postoperative duplex ultrasound evaluates the entire graft, including the anastomoses and perigraft sites, at 1 and 6 months.

In June 1995, we offered a totally laparoscopic ABF bypass to the first patient.[7] The initial approach was not totally satisfactory, and a few days later, the same procedure was performed in a second patient, but under pneumoretroperitoneum. Although the patient did well and was discharged with minimal pain on the fourth postoperative day, the surgical approach to the aorta was again found to be difficult.

PRESENT TECHNIQUE FOR TOTALLY LAPAROSCOPIC AORTOILIAC SURGERY

The operative procedure described below is a laparoscopic abdominal aortic aneurysm resection. A similar approach to the aorta is used for occlusive disease.

Under general anesthesia, and complete hemodynamic monitoring, the patient is positioned supine with a 10° Trendelenburg position and the left side slightly elevated on a pillow. With a Veress needle inserted at the level of the umbilicus, a CO_2 pneumoperitoneum is induced to a maximal pressure of 15 mm Hg. This allows insertion of a 10-mm trocar at the same site, followed by the introduction of a 0° laparoscope (Fig 4, A). One 5-mm trocar and one 10-mm trocar are respectively inserted in the infraumbilical and supraumbilical positions (Fig 4, A). After inspecting the content of the abdominal cavity, the pressure is reduced to 7 mm Hg to facilitate the subsequent retroperitoneal dissection. A 10-mm incision is made 1.5 cm medial and superior to the anterosuperior iliac spine, and the site is sharply dissected to the level of the peritoneum. A finger is then introduced into the retroperitoneal plane to create a small cavity to allow the introduction of the 0° viewing laparoscope. The space is enlarged by dissection with the laparoscope under 15 mm Hg pneumoretroperitoneum (Fig 4, B).

After dissection of the retroperitoneal space, a peritoneal "apron" is created, as previously described,[8] by incising the perito-

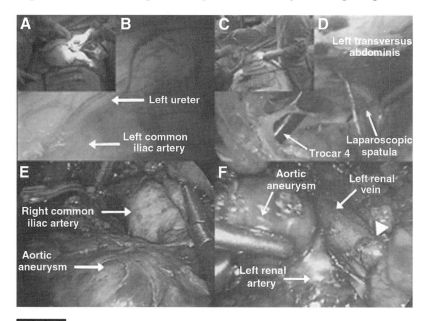

FIGURE 4.
A, Sites of the 7 trocars are depicted. The 3 lateral trocars are placed after the 3 median ones. The last one is inserted in the upper rectus sheath. **B,** Left ureter next to the left common iliac artery is seen as the retroperitoneum is dissected with the laparoscope *(inset)*. **C** and **D,** Peritoneal "apron" is created with a laparoscopic spatula until the previously made posterior retroperitoneal dissection is reached, when *trocar 4* is seen. **E,** Right iliac artery is dissected to its bifurcation. **F,** Visualization of the left renal vein determines the cephalad aspect of the dissection. The gonadal vein is clipped at its origin *(arrowhead)*.

neum lateral to the left rectus muscle and dissecting it with a lapa roscopic spatula until the previously made posterior retroperitoneal dissection is reached (Fig 4, C and D). This "apron" will keep the small bowel and the left colon on the right side of the patient. The last 2 lateral ports (10 mm and 12 mm, respectively) are then placed in the left flank, followed by the upper left transrectus site.

The aneurysmal mass is not dissected on its right lateral aspect. Dissection of the left lateral aspect of the aneurysm is undertaken carefully, beginning at the level of the left iliac artery. The inferior mesenteric artery (IMA) is usually clipped and divided. Then the right iliac artery is dissected to its bifurcation (Fig 4, E). The left ureter is protected during the procedure. As the neck is reached, the gonadal vein is visualized, clipped, and incised. Visualization of the left renal vein determines the cephalad aspect of the dissection (Fig 4, F).

A tube or bifurcated knitted graft is introduced through the lower left lateral trocar into the retroperitoneal cavity. In the case of an ABF bypass, each limb of the graft is tunneled into its respective femoral region by using an especially devised instrument. After systemic heparinization, the distal aorta or the iliac arteries can be interrupted with a laparoscopic GIA-30 (USSC, Norwalk, Conn) or temporarily occluded with intracorporeal clamps in the case of a tube graft. Figure 5, A shows one intracorporeal clamp placed on the left common iliac, one on the right internal, and a third on the right external iliac artery in an open aneurysm repair. Figure 5, B represents a similar clamp being used to occlude the infrarenal aorta during a laparoscopic aneurysm resection.

The neck of the aneurysm is cross-clamped just below the left renal vein with the use of a laparoscopic aortic clamp. The posterior wall of the aorta is dissected, and the lumbar arteries are clipped. A short longitudinal arteriotomy is made in the aneurysm neck. The aneurysm sac is then opened with heavy laparoscopic scissors. The thrombus (Fig 5, C) is placed in an endobag for later removal, and the posterior wall of the aneurysm is inspected to ensure no lumbar back-bleeding. The aneurysm neck is transected, and the proximal anastomosis is initiated posteriorly with two 20-cm 3-0 polypropylene running sutures (Fig 5, D). The 2 running sutures are tied anteriorly as previously described. Surgicel (Ethicon Inc, Somerville, NJ) is applied around the anastomosis, and the proximal clamp is released. Occasionally, extra sutures are needed to repair leaks. Then the distal anastomosis is performed either on the distal aorta (tube graft) or on the femoral arteries (ABF bypass).

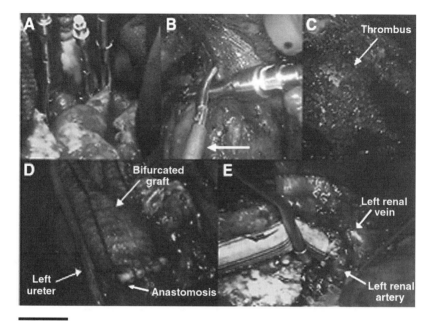

FIGURE 5.
A, Intracorporeal clamps used on the iliac arteries at open surgery. **B,** Similar clamps used during laparoscopic aneurysm resection. A forceps *(arrow)* is used to stabilize the clamp upon removal of the shaft. **C,** Aneurysm sac is opened with heavy laparoscopic scissors, and thrombus is removed with an endobag. **D,** Proximal anastomosis is shown. **E,** Last of the 3 patients with aneurysms larger than 5 cm, who was converted to an assisted laparoscopic procedure for suprarenal clamping and juxtarenal anastomosis. The complete laparoscopic mobilization of the left renal vein allowed for an easy control of the suprarenal aorta during the assisted procedure before performance of a tube graft.

On release of the peritoneal apron, the aneurysm sac and the retroperitoneum cover the graft. The sigmoid colon is inspected. Each of the trocar sites is closed with a single 0-Vicryl suture.

RESULTS

A total of 63 patients were treated. The first 6 received a laparoscopy-assisted ABF bypass, with 3 of them hand assisted. Three patients had a totally laparoscopic iliofemoral bypass, and two additional totally laparoscopic ABF bypasses were done exclusively through the retroperitoneum. We performed our first totally laparoscopic ABF bypass in human beings in 1995, using a gasless, entirely retroperitoneal approach. Because the gasless technique proved difficult, we introduced pneumoperitoneum in the second patient, but performing the entire procedure through the retroperitoneum still remained cumbersome.

In 1996, we suggested a modified transabdominal retroperitoneal approach to reach the aortoiliac segment, an approach that became known as the laparoscopic "apron technique." We describe here our experience with this technique. Forty-nine patients received laparoscopic ABF bypass according to the previously described transabdominal retroperitoneal technique. Table 2 depicts the patients' comorbidity data. To be noted is the presence of severe calcifications (defined as such when concentric) in 21% of the patients (Fig 6).

Indications for surgery were incapacitating claudication in 43 patients, rest pain in 3 patients, and aneurysmal disease in 3 patients. One patient presenting with rest pain had an associated 4.6-cm aortic aneurysm. Major angiographic findings in patients with occlusive disease consisted of total iliac occlusion, severe bilateral iliac stenosis, or recurrent bilateral iliac occlusion after stenting. The average surgery time was 311 minutes (range, 185-510 minutes). The mean aortic crossclamp time was 101 minutes (range, 37-212 minutes), and the mean aortic anastomotic time was 49 minutes (range, 18-155 minutes). The mean blood loss was 686 mL (range, 200-3050 mL), and 7 patients received each 1, 1, 1, 2, 2, 3, and 6 Units of blood.

Six patients required conversion to laparotomy (Table 3). Patient 1 required removal of a plaque fractured at the site of the aortic clamp. Patient 6 bled from an injury to a retroaortic left renal vein, which was controlled laparoscopically. This patient needed replace-

---

TABLE 2.
Preoperative Patient Data

Sex (M/F)	67%/33%
Age (y)	58 (41-76)
Smoking	88%
Hypertension	47%
Myocardial infarction	16%
Angina	9%
Diabetes	9%
ABI right leg	0.67 (0.16-1.10)
ABI left leg	0.63 (0.26-1.06)
Calcifications	Moderate: 41%
	Severe: 21%

Abbreviation: ABI, Ankle-brachial index.

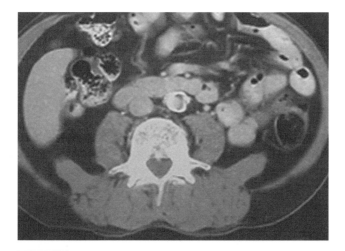

FIGURE 6.

Preoperative computed tomography scan: concentric calcifications of the infrarenal aorta defined as severe.

ment of the graft, which had been damaged during insertion. Patient 7 had an unsatisfactory anastomosis made in a calcified aortic stump. An endarterectomy of the aortic stump was required before a second laparoscopic anastomosis. Patient 40 suddenly developed low blood pressure immediately after thrombectomy of the left leg of the bypass done through the left femoral anastomosis. Since the cause of bleeding was not found after conversion to minilaparotomy because it had stopped, we hypothesized that the Fogarty balloon might have contributed to the bleed by distending the aortic anastomosis. Patient 41 needed conversion because malpositioning prevented an adequate anastomosis. Patient 44 had a juxtarenal aneurysm, and she was aware preoperatively that the totally laparoscopic approach would be used only to facilitate suprarenal clamping, which was performed through a limited laparotomy. Postoperatively, a serious complication occurred in patient 5 who needed a reoperation 3 weeks later for an acute aortic false aneurysm (Table 4). Other complications were caused by a thrombosis of the retroaortic left renal vein after intraoperative ligation and by a prolonged clamping time. One patient who was receiving care on the cardiology floor died of a malignant arrhythmia on the sixth postoperative day. Up to that point, his postoperative course had been entirely satisfactory. One patient treated for an abdominal aortic aneurysm had distal atheromatous emboli from which he recovered without further surgery.

TABLE 3.
Intraoperative Surgical Complications

Patient No.	Complication	Conversion
1	Fractured calcified plaque by crossclamp	Yes (minilap)
6	Bleeding from retroaortic left renal vein, trauma to the graft during insertion	Yes
7	Anastomosis redone laparoscopically after aortic stump endarterectomy	Yes (anastomosis proved adequate)
40	Self-limited bleeding	Yes (minilap)
41	Patient malpositioning, difficult anastomosis	Yes
44	Juxtarenal aneurysm (no complication)	Yes (minilap)

The mean intensive care unit and postoperative hospital stays were 2 days (range, 1-6 days) and 6 days (range, 3-23 days), respectively. All patients who had their bypass done in Quebec have been available for follow-up. All bypasses have been patent. No one needed a reoperation for late thrombosis of the graft. One patient had an ischemic stroke 3 months after surgery.

Most patients were able to take sips of liquid on the first postoperative day and more solid food during the second postoperative day. Postoperative stay is not considered a significant variable since many of our patients live far from the hospital (>650 km). They could have been discharged earlier had they been living within a reasonable distance of Quebec City.

We have treated 6 patients with infrarenal aortic aneurysms, 3 of which were incidental findings during evaluation for occlusive disease. The largest of these 3 measured 4.6 cm and was treated by endoaneurysmorrhaphy with ABF bypass. The 2 others (<4 cm) were excluded during the ABF bypass. Of the 3 remaining patients with aneurysms larger than 5 cm in diameter, 1 underwent Creech's re-

TABLE 4.
Postoperative Complications

Patient No.	Complication	Reoperation
5	Acute aortic false aneurysm	Yes
6	Left renal edema secondary to left retroaortic renal vein thrombosis	No
7	Mild anterior compartment syndrome, right leg	No
20	Sudden death (postop day 6)	No
45	Atheromatous emboli	No
32, 36, 47	Transient hydronephrosis (3 patients)	No

pair associated with an ABF bypass, and a second was managed with an aorto-aortic bypass. The third patient was converted to an assisted laparoscopic procedure for suprarenal clamping and juxtarenal anastomosis. In this case, complete laparoscopic mobilization of the left renal vein allowed for expeditious control of the suprarenal aorta during the assisted procedure before performance of a tube graft (Fig 5, E).

DISCUSSION

When a new technique is developed, one of the initial concerns is the learning curve associated with its application. As already alluded to, laparoscopic aortoiliac surgery is a technique in evolution and, as such, instrumentation has to be developed to facilitate the procedure. Early in our study, we had no laparoscopic instrument dedicated to vascular surgery except an extracorporeal aortic clamp. The technique had to be performed rigorously to avoid potential serious complications. Two experienced vascular and laparoscopic surgeons worked together in each of these procedures. More recently, the technique has been found to be feasible by 1 surgeon assisted with residents, although we suggest that 2 surgeons participate in these procedures.

Suturing is a necessity in laparoscopic surgery. Specific and unique needle drivers have been designed (for both right and left hands) for laparoscopic vascular applications (Fig 7, A and B). They allow for easy handling of sutures such as polypropylene, which has memory, and can manipulate a vascular graft with ease.

Robotic suturing may become an essential part of the laparoscopic vascular surgeon's armamentarium. Systems currently available facilitate the specific task of suturing by providing an excellent 3-dimensional view, coupled with 7° of freedom. As shown in Figure 7, C, distal iliac or aortic anastomoses can be realized from almost any position. Among other instruments useful to achieve a totally laparoscopic bypass, aortic or iliac clamps providing tactile feedback comparable to those used in open procedures were among the first available. Plaque elevators designed for totally laparoscopic endarterectomy and tissue dissection are important components of the instrumentation required (Fig 7, D).

Intracorporeal clamps have recently been made available and have proven helpful during procedures for occlusive aortoiliac disease as well as for infrarenal aneurysm resection. We have tested these clamps in the laboratory and during open surgery, and confirmed their ability to control venous injury to the vena cava or the renal vein. They can be used to clamp the aorta, the iliac arteries, or

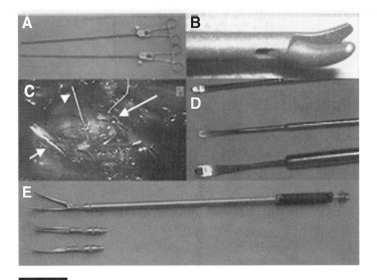

FIGURE 7.

A and **B,** Needle drivers designed for laparoscopic vascular surgery. **C,** Tube grafting done with a robotic system. The distal aortic anastomosis is being performed. The distal aortic clamp is seen to the left of the picture *(short arrow)*. The posterior wall of the anastomosis has been completed, and one arm of the robotic system holds the suture *(arrowhead)*, while the other arm holds the needle that is penetrating the graft *(long arrow)*. **D,** Instruments designed for totally laparoscopic endarterectomy and tissue dissection. **E,** Intracorporeal vascular clamps. Once the distal portion of the clamp is applied on the vessel, the shaft is removed, leaving the trocar site available for other instruments.

any bleeding vessel. As demonstrated in Figure 7, E, the distal portion of the apparatus is the actual vascular clamp, which can be opened and closed on any artery (aorta, iliac, etc). The clamp can be easily affixed to the shaft of the device for either laparoscopic insertion into or removal from the abdominal cavity.

Other useful instruments are the straight and curved DeBakey forceps that can be used to insert the graft or handle vascular tissues. Atraumatic forceps have been designed to safely hold monofilament suture without damage and allow the assistant to follow the running suture. A laparoscopic tunneler was fashioned in such a way as to avoid CO_2 leak from the groins during performance of laparoscopic ABF bypass. Additional instruments include laparoscopic scissors and a laparoscopic nerve hook to tighten the anastomotic suture line.

CONCLUSIONS

For vascular surgeons who have never been exposed to laparoscopy, an assisted approach facilitates the learning curve. Courses are constantly being given on the subject in Quebec and are frequently updated. Advances in instrumentation continue to broaden possible applications. For instance, we have preliminary experience with laparoscopic treatment of endoleaks. Type I endoleaks have been addressed, and a laparoscopic approach could well be offered to those patients whose endoleaks cannot be treated by the endovascular route. Type II endoleaks have also been managed with a laparoscopic approach.

In conclusion, laparoscopic vascular reconstruction has become a feasible alternative in experienced hands. With increased familiarity and improved instrumentation, surgeons should be able to perform these vascular procedures expeditiously and with greater confidence.

REFERENCES

1. Dion YM, Lévesque C, Doillon CJ: Experimental carbon dioxide pulmonary embolization after vena cava laceration under pneumo-peritoneum. *Surg Endosc* 9:1065-1069, 1995.
2. Dion YM, Chin AK, Thompson A: Experimental laparoscopic aortobifemoral bypass. *Surg Endosc* 9:894-897, 1995.
3. Dion YM, Katkhouda N, Rouleau C, et al: Laparoscopy-assisted aortobifemoral bypass. *Surg Laparosc Endosc* 3:425-429, 1993.
4. Dion YM, Gaillard F, Demalsy JC, et al: Experimental laparoscopic aortobifemoral bypass for occlusive aorto-iliac disease. *Can J Surg* 39:451-455, 1996.
5. Dion YM, Gracia CR: A new technique for laparoscopic aortobifemoral grafting in occlusive aortoiliac disease. *J Vasc Surg* 26:685-692, 1997.
6. Dion YM, Gracia CR: Experimental laparoscopic aortic aneurysm resection and aortobifemoral bypass. *Surg Laparosc Endosc* 6:184-190, 1997.
7. Dion YM, Gracia CR, Demalcy JC: Laparoscopic aortic surgery (letter). *J Vasc Surg* 23:539, 1995.
8. Dion YM, Gracia CR, Hartung O: Laparoscopic vascular surgery, in Zucker KA (ed): *Surgical Laparoscopy,* ed 2. Philadelphia, Lippincott Williams & Wilkins, 2000, pp 709-719.

Part III

Peripheral Vascular Disease

CHAPTER 12

Bypass Grafts to the Dorsalis Pedis Artery

Frank W. LoGerfo, MD
William V. McDermott Professor of Surgery, Harvard Medical School,
Chief, Division of Vascular Surgery, Beth Israel Deaconess Medical
Center, Boston, Mass

Establishment of dorsalis pedis bypass as a successful procedure has greatly reduced the incidence of amputations in patients with foot ulcers associated with diabetes mellitus.[1] It may represent the single most important advancement in the care of the diabetic foot since the transmetatarsal amputation.

The complex physiology of foot problems in diabetes creates the setting where extreme distal revascularization, often to the dorsalis pedis artery, is required.[2] It is this physiology that dictates the special considerations necessary in planning and executing arterial reconstruction for maximum success. It is also the physiology that drives the need for multidisciplinary care of these patients.[3] Each of the two primary contributing factors, neuropathy and ischemia, has distinctive characteristics in diabetes.

NEUROPATHY: IMPLICATIONS FOR ARTERIAL RECONSTRUCTION

The polyneuropathy of diabetes has a tendency to compromise the function of the longest, finest nerve fibers first. In terms of motor function, this results in denervation of the intrinsic muscles of the foot, including the lumbrical muscles, which direct the action of the flexor digitorum longus and brevis. Without them, the toes become drawn up in the "claw" position, creating susceptible pressure points on the tips of the toes, the dorsum, especially the proximal interphalangeal joints, and beneath the metatarsal heads. These effects are worsened by the limited joint mobility associated with glycation of scleral proteins. Clawed toes and fixed joints set the stage for pressure ulceration. Although other deformities occur, especially with advanced osteoarthropathy (Charcot foot), the claw foot represents by far the most common deformity as it relates to considerations for arterial reconstruction.

Somatic sensory neuropathy also affects the longest finest nerve fibers (pain and temperature) first. Thus, it is possible for a patient to have relatively intact touch sensation but incur an injury such as stepping on an insulin needle without being aware of it. In addition, there is loss of the nociceptive reflex or neuroinflammatory response.[4] This is the mechanism leading to the "flare" response to a skin injury. It involves the release of neuropeptides and cytokines to cause vasodilatation, increased capillary permeability, and leukocyte migration. Absence of this first-line defense may explain the "masked" response of the foot to infection.

Autonomic neuropathy results in loss of sweat (eccrine) and oil (apocrine) gland function leading to dry skin that easily cracks, creating a portal of entry for infection. Autonomic neuropathy also results in arteriovenous shunting and inefficient perfusion of the capillary bed.

COMPROMISED BIOLOGY: AN IMPORTANT CONCEPT

In addition to the well-documented and visible effects of neuropathy, there are less specific effects of diabetes, such as the glycation of proteins, that probably add to the compromised biology of the foot

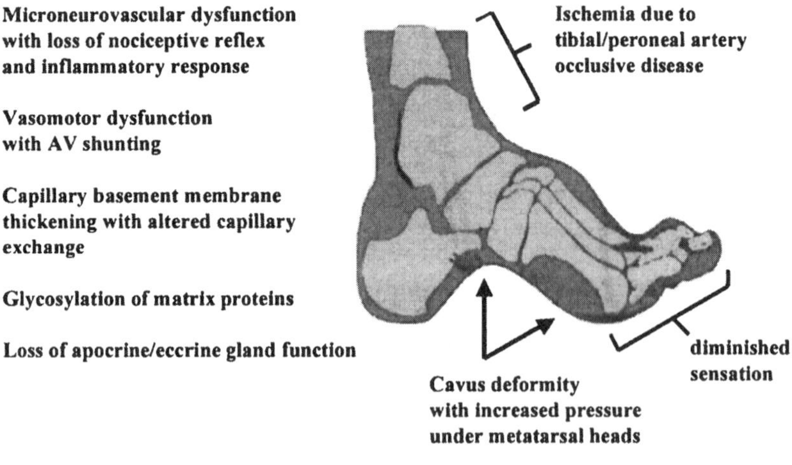

Microneurovascular dysfunction with loss of nociceptive reflex and inflammatory response

Vasomotor dysfunction with AV shunting

Capillary basement membrane thickening with altered capillary exchange

Glycosylation of matrix proteins

Loss of apocrine/eccrine gland function

Ischemia due to tibial/peroneal artery occlusive disease

Cavus deformity with increased pressure under metatarsal heads

diminished sensation

FIGURE 1.

Pathophysiology of the diabetic foot leading to ulceration, tissue loss, or both. *Abbreviation: AV,* Arteriovenous.

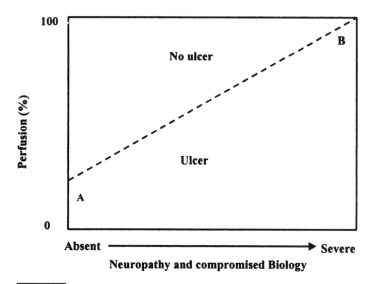

FIGURE 2.
The diagram illustrates the relationship between ulceration, compromised biology, and ischemia. When ischemia is severe, even a foot with perfect biology will ulcerate *(point A)*. With severe neuropathy and compromised biology, even a well-perfused foot will ulcerate *(point B)*. All patients are somewhere between these two extremes. Even when biology is significantly compromised, an improvement in perfusion will result in healing of the ulcer, healing of minor amputations and debridements, or both.

(Fig 1). At its worst, neuropathy and compromised biology can lead to ulceration of the foot, even with perfectly intact circulation. In the absence of any neuropathy or compromised biology, the foot is highly resistant to pressure ulceration, even with severe ischemia. All patients are somewhere between these extremes. As neuropathy increases, it takes increased perfusion to maintain an intact foot. This can be illustrated graphically (Fig 2).

ISCHEMIA IN THE DIABETIC FOOT

In spite of an entrenched misconception, there are no data to support the existence of a small vessel or microcirculatory occlusion in the diabetic foot.[5] Although the capillary basement membrane is thickened, the capillary lumen is not narrowed.[6] Thus, arterial reconstruction to an artery in continuity to the foot will be effective in restoring tissue perfusion.

The pattern of atherosclerotic occlusive disease in diabetes tends to involve the infrageniculate arteries but with relative spar-

Ing of the arteries in the foot, especially the dorsalis pedis.[7] Because of the compromised biology, it is desirable to restore maximum perfusion to the diabetic foot. Often, in about 30% of our patients with diabetes mellitus and foot lesions, the dorsalis pedis is the only target that can provide direct perfusion of the foot. If the anterior or posterior tibial arteries are patent into the foot, they are equivalently effective targets. The peroneal artery, however, is not in direct continuity and is not an equivalently effective target. The peroneal is a suitable second choice when for some reason, usually conduit limitations, the dorsalis pedis cannot be used.

Inflow to the bypass can be from the most distal artery proximal to which there is no significant stenosis. For patients with occlusive disease involving both the superficial femoral and infrageniculate arteries, the common femoral artery must be used. When only the infrageniculate arteries are occluded, the distal popliteal is the first choice.

ARTERIOGRAPHY

Accurate detailed arteriography is essential to planning and executing any distal bypass, with some special considerations for dorsalis pedis bypass. The most reliable current technique is digital subtraction arteriography. The key views are the anteroposterior and the lateral projections of the foot. These should include the toes so that choices between targets can be based on best perfusion of the area of the foot lesion. When positioning the patient for these studies, the foot should not be taped or held down in plantar flexion because this may cause "pseudo-occlusion" of the dorsalis pedis where it passes over the navicular bone. If the catheter is placed in the opposite common femoral artery and passed across the aortic bifurcation, it can be easily positioned in the ipsilateral common femoral or superficial femoral artery. From this position, excellent runoff views can be obtained with minimal contrast agent. In patients with elevated serum creatinine levels in whom there is concern about the use of iodinated contrast agents, carbon dioxide can be used for the aortoiliac segments. Along with pullout pressures, this will provide sufficient information about inflow to make informed decisions in planning the operative procedure, and limit the volume of contrast agent to 30 to 40 mL.

EXPOSURE OF THE DORSALIS PEDIS ARTERY

The dorsalis pedis artery is usually located just under the lateral margin of the extensor hallucis longus tendon. If there is any question with regard to topographic anatomy, a Doppler can be used as a guide in marking the skin. This will help avoid undermining of the skin or excessive retraction. The incision is then made directly over the course of the artery in its most proximal segment at the origin of the medial and lateral tarsal arteries, requiring division of a portion of the extensor retinaculum.

The artery is usually somewhat calcified. With a forceps, the artery can be palpated to identify the softest area for anastomosis. In those unusual instances where the artery is completely pipelike with calcification, intraluminal vessel occluders have been helpful. We have noted only a minor decrease in patency when the vessel was so calcified that the intraluminal occluders were necessary.[8] Tourniquets have not been successful in providing arterial occlusion in patients with severely calcified arteries, in our experience.

Anastomosis is carried out with standard loupes and 6-0 or 7-0 Prolene. The main difficulty encountered is with calcification. When the needle will not pass through a calcification, it is helpful to wiggle the tip of the needle against the arterial wall for several seconds and usually it will pass through. Sometimes 2 or 3 sutures will be placed that incorporate only adventitia. Surprisingly, this is usually successful provided there are several sutures on each side that incorporate the full thickness of the arterial wall. The important message here is that even calcified arteries should be regarded as suitable targets provided an adequate lumen has been documented by arteriography.

INCISIONS, TUNNELING, AND SKIN CLOSURE

Many of these patients are obese, and incisions that cross the groin crease can be problematic. If a segment of superficial femoral artery is patent, it is advantageous to use this for the proximal anastomosis to avoid the need to cross the groin crease with an incision.

When using the in situ technique, we use 2 parallel incisions on the foot. This provides maximum latitude for identifying a target site on the dorsalis pedis and for mobilizing an adequate segment of distal vein. As a result, there is a skin bridge between the 2 incisions, and it is important to avoid tunneling the graft under this bridge. The subcutaneous tunnel should pass proximal to this (Fig 3).

When using the popliteal artery for inflow, it is possible to harvest the vein beginning above the ankle to avoid the parallel incisions, although this is not as important as avoiding the tunnel under the skin bridge (Fig 4). Vein grafts from the popliteal may be reversed, nonreversed, arm vein,[9] lesser saphenous, etc. It is preferable to tunnel this graft beneath the superficial fascia to the lower leg and then subcutaneously anterior to the tibia to reach the dorsalis pedis.

Marginal necrosis of wound edges is not uncommon in patients with diabetes. This is worrisome when it occurs over grafts in the in situ position and, especially, at the distal incision over the dorsalis pedis anastomosis. Closure of the distal incisions warrants some extra attention to minimize this problem. My preference is to close the subcutaneous tissue with interrupted absorbable suture and to use interrupted 3-0 nylon for the skin. Alternatives, such as subcuticular skin closure with or without adhesive strips, are equally effective. Caution is advised with regard to using skin staples, as they tend to gather in skin and are not as controllable as sutures in preventing undo tension or achieving accurate wound edge approximation.

Postreconstruction edema, probably enhanced by the albumin capillary leak of diabetes, may add to wound tension on the ankle and foot. Wrapping the foot and ankle with elastic bandage, leaving

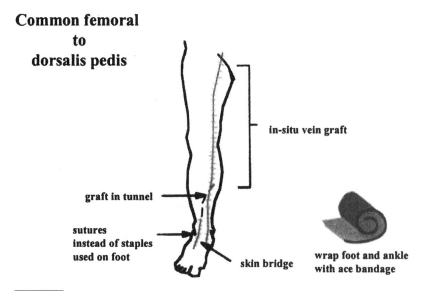

FIGURE 3.

When inflow is from the common femoral artery, the in situ technique is preferred. It is important to tunnel the graft above the skin bridge, to not use staples for closure of the foot wounds, and to use an elastic bandage or elevation to minimize swelling and stress on the suture line.

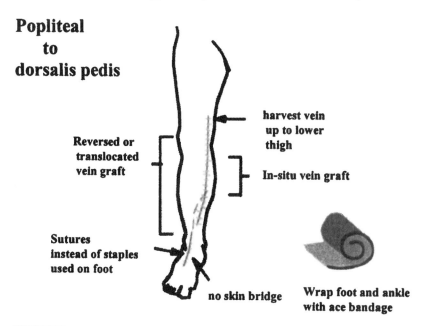

Popliteal to dorsalis pedis

harvest vein up to lower thigh

Reversed or translocated vein graft

In-situ vein graft

Sutures instead of staples used on foot

no skin bridge

Wrap foot and ankle with ace bandage

FIGURE 4.

When inflow is from the popliteal artery, the translocated or reversed technique is preferred. This eliminates the skin bridge and makes it possible to position the graft underneath the fascia for most of its length.

a small port for palpation of the distal grafts, is effective in limiting the swelling. Alternatively, the foot may be well elevated on pillows.

PERIOPERATIVE CARE

Virtually all patients undergoing these procedures have coronary artery disease. We have not performed routine stress testing, although most of our patients have an echocardiogram to determine left ventricular function. On the other hand, we carefully monitor patients, most of whom have a pulmonary artery catheter, and all have central venous pressure monitoring. Infusion of intravenous fluids is limited as much as possible during the operation. Typically, patients receive 1200 mL of intravenous fluid during a 3-hour operation with about 200 mL of blood loss. This is distinctly different from patients undergoing laparotomy where the fluid requirements are higher, a point that must be made for anesthesiologists. Most of our patients receive general anesthesia, since there is no difference in outcome with spinal or epidural anesthesia.[10]

Postoperatively, patients are observed in an intermediate care unit with central monitoring until their fluid balance is restored. When body weight is at or near preoperative weight, monitoring is discontinued. For most patients this requires 2 postoperative days. In general, our management of coronary artery disease emphasizes close monitoring during the perioperative period, with less emphasis on preoperative studies, especially routine stress testing or cardiac catheterization. We have not found diabetes mellitus to be an independent risk factor for perioperative myocardial infarction or death.[11]

If these guidelines are followed, vein grafts to the dorsalis pedis artery can be performed with a very low mortality rate and an expectation of success similar to that of other infrageniculate bypass grafts. In more than 1000 vein bypass grafts to the dorsalis pedis artery, our 30-day operative mortality rate is 0.97% and 5-year primary assisted patency rate is 62%, with limb salvage at 78%.[12]

CONCLUSION

Vein grafts to the dorsalis pedis artery can be performed with a very low mortality rate and a patency rate similar to that of other infrageniculate bypass grafts. The operation is especially appropriate for many patients with diabetes mellitus and foot ulcers when ischemia is a contributing factor. Flexibility in the choice of inflow site, graft preparation, tunneling, and skin closure contributes to success. Perioperative cardiac care should be designed to avoid excessive intravenous fluid administration and heart failure.

REFERENCES

1. LoGerfo FW, Gibbons GW, Pomposelli FB Jr, et al: Trends in the care of the diabetic foot. Expanded role of arterial reconstruction. *Arch Surg* 127:617-621, 1992.
2. LoGerfo FW: The diabetic foot, in Cameron JL (ed): *Current Surgical Therapy*. St Louis, Mosby, 1995, pp 746-748.
3. Veves A, Giurini JM, LoGerfo FW: *The Diabetic Foot*. Totawa, NJ, Humana Press, 2001.
4. Walmsley D, Wiles PG: Early loss of neurogenic inflammation in the human diabetic foot. *Clin Sci* 80:605-610, 1991.
5. LoGerfo FW, Coffman JD: Vascular and microvascular disease of the foot in diabetes: Implications for foot care. *N Engl J Med* 311:1615-1619, 1984.
6. Siperstein MD, Unger RH, Madison LL: Studies of muscle capillary basement membranes in normal subjects, diabetic, and prediabetic patients. *J Clin Invest* 47:1973-1999, 1968.

7. Menzoian JO, LaMorte WW, Paniszyn CC, et al: Symptomatology and anatomic patterns of peripheral vascular disease: Differing impact of smoking and diabetes. *Ann Vasc Surg* 3:224-228, 1989.

8. Misare BD, Pomposelli FB Jr, Gibbons GW, et al: Infrapopliteal bypasses to severely calcified, unclampable outflow arteries: Two year results. *J Vasc Surg* 24:6-16, 1996.

9. Pomposelli FB Jr, Marcaccio E, Gibbons GW, et al: Dorsalis pedis arterial bypass: Durable limb salvage for foot ischemia in patients with diabetes mellitus. *J Vasc Surg* 21:375-384, 1995.

10. Pierce ET, Pomposelli FB Jr, Stanley GD, et al: Anesthesia type does not influence early graft patency or limb salvage rates of lower extremity arterial bypass. *J Vasc Surg* 25:226-232, 1997.

11. Hamdan AD, Satzberg SS, Sheahan M, et al: 6565 major vascular operations: Diabetes is not associated with increased postoperative mortality and cardiac morbidity. *Arch Surg*, in press.

12. Pomposelli FB, LoGerfo FW, Hamdan A: Outcome of 1037 bypass grafts to the dorsalis pedis artery. *J Vasc Surg*, in press.

CHAPTER 13

Saphenous Vein Allografts for Infrainguinal Arterial Reconstruction: Current Role as Vascular Conduits

Carlos H. Timaran, MD

Chief Resident, Department of Surgery, University of Tennessee Medical Center, Knoxville

Mitchell H. Goldman, MD

Professor and Chairman, Department of Surgery, University of Tennessee Medical Center, Knoxville

Autologous saphenous vein is the graft of choice for patients who require lower extremity revascularization.[1,2] When greater saphenous veins are unsuitable or have been previously harvested, lesser saphenous or arm veins can be used with acceptable results.[3] Alternative grafts, in the absence of a suitable autologous vein for reconstruction, such as prosthetic grafts and arterial allografts, have been used with poor results.[2,4] In addition, arterial allografts have been associated with early rupture and aneurysmal degeneration.[5] Thus, the concept and potential utility of vein allografts from cadaver donors stems from the need for alternative conduits for infrainguinal arterial reconstruction in patients with limb-threatening ischemia and extensive femoropopliteal occlusive disease who lack autologous veins. Otherwise, these patients would undergo amputation, procedures with prosthetic grafts, or expectant treatment for limb-threatening ischemia.

Cryopreserved vein allografts have been used for infrainguinal arterial reconstruction, hemodialysis access, and more recently, as a potential source for replacement of dysfunctional valves in the treatment of chronic venous insufficiency.[6-10] Moreover, cryopreserved veins or veins from cadaver sources have been used in infected fields where autologous veins are unavailable.[11] Despite early purported success, long-term results have not been encouraging, and the role of vein allografts remains undefined.[12] Sustained immunogenic activity, rejection, and loss of endothelial lining associated with cryopreserved allografts have been considered as probable causes of failure.[6-8,13,14] Immunosuppression and anticoagulation, as well as improvement in harvesting techniques and use of cryopreservants with controlled freezing, have been used to improve allograft patency.[15,16] The use of cryopreserved vein allografts has clear advantages: off-the-shelf availability, and therefore reduced operating and anesthesia time; and limited incisions and reduced wound complications, which usually allow early ambulation and reduced length of hospital stay.

Allograft conduits that are not immunogenic would be ideal for infrainguinal bypass procedures. Greater saphenous veins obtained from cadavers and preserved by lyophilization are an attractive source of venous allografts for arterial reconstructions. The freeze-drying process renders the tissue nonimmunogenic.[17] After reconstitution, lyophilized vessels demonstrate handling characteristics similar to fresh veins.[18] In previous experimental studies, lyophilized allografts have demonstrated patency and structural integrity in both the arterial and venous systems.[17]

Arterial allografts have been recently reconsidered for lower extremity revascularization in Europe.[4] Long-term results reveal acceptable limb salvage but poor allograft patency. Aneurysmal degeneration, although less frequent with new methods of cryopreservation, continue to be a matter of concern. The only commercially prepared arterial allografts available in the United States are aortoiliac allografts used for replacement of infected aortic grafts and treatment of mycotic aneurysms.

TECHNIQUE OF CRYOPRESERVATION

Several cryopreservation techniques have being introduced to attain the best method for proper procurement, cryoprotection, freezing, storage, and thawing, thereby preserving functional and structural characteristics of the native vein. The ideal method for developing the perfect vein allograft, however, has not been found. It is unclear whether the presence of viable and functional allogenic cells in cryopreserved vein allografts is beneficial. Nevertheless, the main objective of cryopreservation of tissues from cadaver donors is to obtain minimal antigenic allografts with optimal functional and structural integrity. The American Association of Tissue Banks and the United Network for Organ Sharing have established standards and requirements for tissue preservation. Organ procurement agencies, such as CryoLife Inc (Kennesaw, Ga) and Norwest Tissue Center (Seattle, Wash), provide cryopreserved vein allografts for vascular reconstruction. Although no known cases of viral or bacterial transmission with the transplantation of cryopreserved allografts have been reported, all donors are carefully screened and tested by using the Centers for Disease Control and Prevention criteria for viral, bacterial, and fungal communicable diseases. The effect of cryopreservation on viral and bacterial inactivation is unknown, but theoretically, a small risk of viral transmission exists.

Saphenous veins are harvested from cadaver donors within 24 hours after circulatory arrest. Meticulous atraumatic surgical technique is necessary to preserve the functional and structural integrity of the vein graft. According to one of the manufacturers (CryoLife, Inc), veins are harvested with a "no touch" technique and kept moist with medium, which contains 10% bovine serum and papaverine, 0.12 mg/mL. The allograft is then stored in vapor of liquid nitrogen between $-110°C$ and $-196°C$ by using cryoprotectants, which prevent the formation of an intracellular vapor gradient and lethal intracellular ice crystals that could lead to cellular membrane disruption during the freezing process and thawing, thereby affecting the integrity of cells of the vein graft. Dimethyl sulfoxide (DMSO), in 10% or 20% concentration, and chondroitin sulfate are the most commonly used cryoprotectants. Without cryoprotectants, the use of saphenous vein allografts has been associated with high graft failure rates after infrainguinal bypass procedures.[19]

PHYSIOLOGY AND IMMUNOLOGY OF CRYOPRESERVED VEIN ALLOGRAFTS

In experimental studies, cryopreservation has been proved to preserve many potentially beneficial functional features of both endothelial and smooth muscle cells including prostacyclin and endothelin production, fibrinolytic activity, thrombotic properties, metabolic mechanisms, and to some extent, elasticity, contractility, and compliance.[20] Morphologic characteristics are also maintained. In preserving such desirable properties, however, immunogenicity is also retained, and the immune response to venous allografts has been shown to play a fundamental role in ultimate graft patency.[14]

Several experimental and clinical studies have shown almost immediate endothelial denudation of cryopreserved vein allografts after implantation in arterial circuits.[13,14] The allografted endothelium is sheared off early and is subsequently replaced by autogenous endothelial cells.[21] Such loss of endothelium is probably related to the inability of current methods of cryopreservation to maintain cellular adherence. It is unlikely that endothelial washout is the result of an immune phenomenon. The denuded endothelial cells, however, are still antigenic and may serve as sources of antigen-presenting cells.[14] The ultimate immune response may then be directed against smooth muscle cells, thereby contributing to the development of intimal hyperplasia and subsequent late graft failure. In this regard, experimental studies have demonstrated a decreased relaxation response of cryopreserved smooth muscle cells to nitric oxide, phenylephrine, and endothelin.[19] Such decreased contractile response may be caused in part by cellular damage of allografted smooth muscle cells after cryopreserved vein implantation. According to a recent study, endothelial and smooth cells of recipient origin repopulate the endothelial layer and vessel wall of cryopreserved vein allografts, thereby resulting in a completely renewed cellular conduit or a mosaic of host and donor cells.[21] The loss of donor cells may be mediated by apoptosis or rejection. Immunosuppression did not appear to affect the degree of cellular repopulation. The functional features of the repopulated allograft and its neoendothelium and their influence on maintenance of allograft patency are unknown. Cryopreserved vein allografts may be more thrombogenic during the interval before the replacement of the endothelium. Therefore, the use of antiplatelet agents and anticoagulants is justified early after implantation.

Although it was initially considered that cryopreserved venous allografts were either nonantigenic or only weakly antigenic, recent studies have demonstrated that venous tissue expresses class I and II major histocompatibility complex (MHC) antigens and non-MHC antigens that stimulate a T cell–mediated rejection response.[14,21] Cryopreservation does not significantly affect this antigenicity. Cellular infiltrates have been demonstrated in all explanted cryopreserved allografts. Most inflammatory cells have proved to be activated T cells, expressing CD3, CD8, and HLA-DR antigens. The presence of this infiltrate correlates with vessel wall hemorrhage and necrosis. The immune-mediated inflammatory response secondary to rejection combined with cryopreservation and surgical injuries and rheologic mismatch may compound and accelerate the development of intimal hyperplasia and lead to allograft failure. In addition to cellular immunity, vein allografts have also been proved to induce the development of anti-HLA antibodies after bypass allografting, suggesting an associated humoral immune response.[13] These anti-HLA antibodies may contribute to allograft failure by enhancing opsonization of venous allograft antigens, leading to activation of the complement cascade, and facilitating the cellular immune response mediated by cytotoxic T cells. Because of the limited availability of vein allografts, HLA matching is not feasible for clinical applications, and only ABO compatibility has been evaluated in most studies. The role of ABO and HLA matching for human beings has not been determined.

Rejection does not only play a significant role in venous allograft failure, but leads to allosensitization. Benedetto et al[22] noted that implantation of cryopreserved saphenous vein grafts for hemodialysis access causes allosensitization with increased alloantibody production, as measured by elevated panel reactivity antibody levels. Furthermore, the authors found that this allosensitization prevented these patients with chronic renal failure from undergoing kidney transplantation. What appeared to be a potential advantage of the use of DMSO as the cryopreservant (ie, the availability of cryopreserved tissue with retained functional cellular elements) led to allosensitization in these nonimmunosuppressed patients. The exposure to allogenic MHC and non-MHC antigens present on the cryopreserved endothelial cell is postulated as the mechanism of allosensitization. To prevent such immunologic activation and rejection, a new cryopreserved femoral vein allograft has been introduced (CryoVein SG, Cryolife, Inc). The donor endothelial cells present in the allograft are enzymatically removed, whereas the collagen matrix is maintained, theoretically allowing the recipient's endothelial cells to seed the allograft. To some extent, progress has taken us back to the beginning when the main concern was to decrease the thombogenicity of cryopreserved vein allografts related to the loss of endothelial cells secondary to the action of cryopreservants. A multicenter prospective clinical trial is underway to evaluate the use of endothelium-depleted cryopreserved vein allografts for hemodialysis access and its effects on allosensitization and graft patency.

Lamm et al[23] recently reported the use of deendothelialized cryopreserved vein allografts seeded with autologous endothelial cells (ie, the recipient's own venous endothelial cells) before implantation for coronary artery bypass grafting procedures in human beings. This is the first report to document the use of autologous endothelialized vein allografts for any type of arterial reconstruction in human beings and suggests that these allografts offer clinical safety and may be easily developed. In contrast to other tissue-

engineered grafts, the average production period of this new al
lograft was only 3 weeks. After histologic and biomechanical tests
and quality assessment of the new grafts were obtained, 12 patients
receive 15 allografts. Two occlusions had occurred at the first coronary angiographic follow-up. Although the initial clinical results
with this new tissue-engineered alternative allograft appear promis-
ing, the follow-up period of this study is still limited (the oldest allograft has been implanted for about 3 years). These preliminary results should promote further study of this recently developed
autologous endothelialized allograft and its potential use for peripheral reconstructions.

CLINICAL USE AND RESULTS

Currently, cryopreserved saphenous vein allografts can be obtained
through several commercial companies and ordered overnight to
any hospital in the United States. Human greater saphenous veins
for cryopreservation are obtained from cadaver donors who had no
known history of venous insufficiency or venous thrombosis.
Matching for ABO blood type and Rh compatibility is recommended
to prevent an immune response between the recipient and the allogenic graft. To maintain cellular viability, cryopreserved vein allografts should be stored in dry ice packing and only for up to 72
hours. When ready for usage, the vein allograft is initially sub-
merged in a warm water bath (37°C to 42°C) that thaws the vein allograft, preserving cellular viability. Before implantation, the allograft is further prepared with different solutions provided by the
vendor. After reconstitution, cryopreserved vein allografts demonstrate near-ideal sewing and handling characteristics very similar to
those of fresh veins. Most vein allografts average 3.5 to 5.5 mm in
diameter. Intravenous heparin is administered for systemic anticoagulation before vascular clamping. Irrigation of the cryopreserved
vein with heparinized saline solution is important to determine the
antegrade flow direction of the vein allograft.

Since the early work of Yamanouchi in 1911, Carrell in 1912,
and the first implantation of a saphenous vein allograft in human
beings for an arterial bypass reconstruction in 1955 by Shaw and
Wheelock, several series in which cryopreserved vein allografts
were used have been published.[19] Because of adverse results obtained with the first cryopreserved vein allografts available, the en-
thusiasm for the use of this alternative allograft waned. In recent
years, however, cryopreserved saphenous vein allografts have been
used more frequently. Renewed interest in these allografts stems
from new methods of cryopreservation and controlled freezing, the

use of immunosuppression and anticoagulation, as well as the improvement in harvesting techniques.

Since more uniform techniques for cryopreservation were introduced, series with vein allografts obtained from similar commercial sources have been published (Table 1). Before this, reports did not adhere to current reporting standards[24] and methods of cryopreservation, and therefore were difficult to interpret. All series were retrospective and therefore subjected to the limitations of this type of review. In addition, initial studies only included short-term results, and therefore no conclusive evidence about the outcome of these conduits was available. Harris et al[6] reported a secondary patency rate of 36% at 1 year in a study of 25 infrainguinal arterial reconstructions. Walker et al[7] found primary patency rates of 28% at 12 months and 14% at 18 months, in a series of 39 lower extremity arterial reconstructions. Secondary patency rates were 46 and 37%, respectively. Poor results in these 2 series can be explained, as most vein allografts were used for secondary procedures with distal anastomoses in infrageniculate vessels. In addition, Walker et al also used composite grafts in 40% of their procedures with adjunctive synthetic materials. Shah et al[8] published more favorable results,

TABLE 1.

Infrainguinal Arterial Reconstructions With Cryopreserved Saphenous Vein Allografts

Study	Year	No. of Allografts	Patency Rates* (%)				Limb Salvage (%)			
			1 y	2 y	3 y	4 y	1 y	2 y	3 y	4 y
Harris et al[6]	1993	25	36†	—	—	—	74	—	—	—
Walker et al[7]	1993	39	28	—	—	—	67	—	—	—
Shah et al[8]	1993	43	66	53	—	—	—	—	—	—
Martin et al[25]	1994	115	37	19	9	3	84	81	—	62
Posner et al[15]	1996	21	59‡	—	—	—	—	—	—	—
Leseche et al[26]	1997	25	52†	—	—	—	—	78	—	—
Carpenter and Tomaszewski[13]	1998	40	13	13	—	—	42	42	—	—
Cryolife volunteer registry	1998	381	38	28	23	22	73	72	70	70
Buckley et al[16]	2000	26	87	82	—	—	88	80	—	—
Harris et al[12]	2001	80	37	32	24	—	66	62	62	—

*All rates denote primary patency unless indicated.
†Only secondary patency rates reported in the study.
‡Primary patency in patients who received cyclosporine (vs 36% in patients who did not receive it).

with a 00% cumulative patency rate at 1 year. Most procedures were primary reconstructions (55%) with distal anastomosis in the popliteal artery (60%). Multivariate logistic regression analysis revealed that primary reconstructions, compared with reoperations, and the use of one segment of vein allograft were independent predictors for improved graft patency. Postoperative anticoagulation with warfarin did not influence allograft patency in any of these 3 series, but because a retrospective analysis was used in these studies, this finding may be inaccurate. Because endothelial properties were mostly preserved, the inadequacy of structural and functional media characteristics, such as elasticity and compliance, of the cryopreserved vein allograft were suggested as the cause of the adverse results and the tendency of some grafts toward aneurysmal degeneration.

Martin et al[25] have reported the largest series of cryopreserved saphenous vein allografts implanted for lower extremity arterial revascularization, with 115 vein allografts implanted in 87 limbs. The follow-up period was 25 months, with a range between 1 and 61 months. Tibial arteries (88%) were the primary sites of distal anastomoses, and 80% of procedures were performed for limb salvage. Despite controlled freezing and the use of DMSO, primary patency rates at 1, 2, and 4 years were only 37%, 19%, and 3%, respectively, whereas secondary patency rates were 40%, 28%, and 11%, respectively. In contrast, limb salvage rates at 1, 2, and 4 years were 84%, 81%, and 62%, respectively. Immunosuppression was not used in this series. Anticoagulation with warfarin or aspirin had no significant effect on allograft failure. In only 4 patients with allograft failure and thrombosis was histologic examination obtained. No evidence of rejection or immune response was evident. In 6 patients, allograft revision was required for aneurysmal dilatation. Based on their findings, the authors concluded that although satisfactory limb salvage is feasible, long-term patency rates for cryopreserved vein allografts are poor. When compared with prosthetic grafts and according to concurrent published data, cryopreserved veins offered comparable or inferior results at a far higher cost. Moreover, long-term integrity and aneurysmal dilatation were another concern with vein allografts. In the authors' view, cryopreserved vein allografts should be reserved for patients without suitable autogenous veins and a high risk of infection that precludes the use of prosthetic grafts.

Leseche et al[26] performed a prospective study of 25 patients undergoing femorodistal bypass procedures with cryopreserved vein allografts for limb salvage. The secondary patency rate was 52% at 1 year, and the limb salvage rate was 78% at 2 years. Duplex ultrasound was used for allograft surveillance and allowed the early identification and repair of several abnormalities before graft failure, with no increased morbidity or mortality. However, a high frequency of allograft thrombosis occurred during the first postoperative year at a time when no underlying previous graft lesion had been identified with duplex surveillance scan. These authors also reported improved cryopreserved vein allograft patency by the use of postoperative anticoagulation with low molecular weight heparin and aspirin therapy.

Because cryopreservation does not affect allograft antigenicity, immunosuppression has been used as a possible means to improve allograft patency of cryopreserved veins. However, contradictory results have been reported regarding the beneficial effects of adjunctive immunosuppression on allograft patency. In animal studies, immunosuppression has been shown to improve cryopreserved allograft patency, whereas in human beings no clear benefit has been observed.[13,15] Sample sizes in these clinical studies, however, have been small, and hence, the possibility of a type II statistical error is significant. Posner et al[15] noted significantly improved actuarial 12-month primary patency of cryopreserved vein allografts used for infrainguinal arterial reconstructions when immunosuppression with low-dose cyclosporine, azathioprine, and prednisone was instituted in combination with vasodilators and anticoagulants (aspirin and warfarin). These authors, however, also had a substantial number of allograft-related complications including early degeneration, pseudoaneurysm formation, and hemorrhage. Conversely, in the only randomized prospective clinical trial of the use of cryopreserved vein allografts for infrainguinal bypass procedures, Carpenter and Tomaszewski[13] found that low-dose immunosuppression with azathioprine did not affect primary patency and limb salvage. In a companion study,[14] the authors postulated that vein allograft failure is not only mediated by rejection, which is not eliminated by low-dose azathioprine, but also by local injury, hypercoagulability, or stasis. More potent immunosuppression and anticoagulation were suggested as means of mitigating the contribution of rejection and local hypercoagulability to venous allograft failure. Immunosuppression, therefore, has improved cryopreserved vein allograft patency only in animal models, and has improved human arterial allograft patency in transplant recipients when high-dose immunosuppression is instituted.[15,19] In the clinical setting, immunosuppression has not proved effective in arterial reconstructions with vein allografts, in part because the low-dose immunosuppression regimens used do not reach the level of suppression obtained in clinical transplantation to curtail the allogenic response. More potent immunosuppression, however, may not be appropriate because of several reasons: the toxicity of available medications, which may not be tolerated by older patients with multiple comorbidities; the risk of infection, especially in patients with tissue loss; and the failure to improve allograft patency of cryopreserved veins used in liver transplantation.[27] Moreover, in a recent study from our institution, histologic and immunohistochemical analyses of renal arterial allografts of failed transplant kidneys were performed in patients who required transplant nephrectomy. Evidence of chronic rejection and intimal hyperplasia was noted in all major vessel walls. All of these patients had received high-dose immunosuppression, which did not prevent rejection.

Harris et al[12] published recently one of the few studies with long-term results. In their study, 76 patients underwent 80 cryopreserved vein bypass-grafting procedures for limb salvage. The long-term allograft patency rate was 24% at 3 years, with a 62% rate of limb salvage. The authors noted that additional attempts at revascularization for failed grafts did not result in improved long-term limb salvage. Finally, skin integrity was a significant concern in this series. Ulceration either persisted or recurred in 55% of patients available for follow-up, raising doubts about the long-term efficacy of infrainguinal reconstructions with cryopreserved veins. Although the study included only bypass-grafting procedures with vein allografts and therefore no direct comparison with prosthetic grafts was performed, the authors suggested considering the use of polytetrafluoroethylene grafts with adjunctive patches or cuffs rather than implanting cryopreserved veins.

Buckley et al[16] prospectively assessed an anticoagulation protocol to improve allograft patency and limb salvage in patients undergoing femoral-infrapopliteal bypass reconstructions with cryopreserved vein allografts in a recent cohort study. The protocol included the perioperative administration of low-dose heparin and low molecular weight dextran 40 intravenous infusions, and the postoperative use of low-dose aspirin (81 mg/d), dipyridamole (75 mg twice a day), and warfarin (to a therapeutic international normalized ratio of 2.0-2.5). Immunosuppressive agents were not used. During a 4-year period, 24 patients underwent 26 lower extremity bypass grafting procedures for limb salvage. A concurrent control group of patients was not provided; therefore, the conclusions were based on assumptions after comparing the results of the study with recently published data. Primary allograft patency was 82% at 2 years, and the limb salvage rate was 80%. The treatment protocol, according to the authors, substantially improved allograft patency and limb salvage when compared with data provided by recent studies and the manufacturer (CryoLife, Inc) (Figs 1 and 2). Without an independent placebo-controlled group of similar patients, it is not clear whether the improved outcome in this series is the result of the experimental treatment or some other factors. This study also analyzed several disadvantages associated with the use of cryopreserved vein allografts. Anticoagulation had to be discontinued in 3 patients (12%) because of gastrointestinal bleeding. A limited cost analysis was also made and revealed that cryopreserved veins were not only expensive but caused significant losses and, therefore, were not cost-effective. The cost for each allograft used in this series oscillated between $4200 and $4600, whereas total hospital expenses per case ranged from $13,730 to $17,341. Only during the last year of the study were costs reduced to the point of breaking even, in part

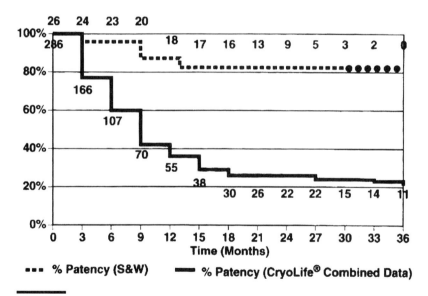

FIGURE 1.

Primary patency curves of femoral-infrapopliteal bypass grafting procedures with Cryo-Vein (CryoLife) allografts as reported by Buckley et al[16] (S & W) in their study and outlined in the CryoLife registry. *Abbreviation: S & W,* Scott & White Clinic. (Courtesy of Buckley CJ, Abernathy S, Lee SD, et al: Suggested treatment protocol for improving patency of femoral-infrapopliteal cryopreserved saphenous vein allografts. *J Vasc Surg* 32:731-738, 2000.)

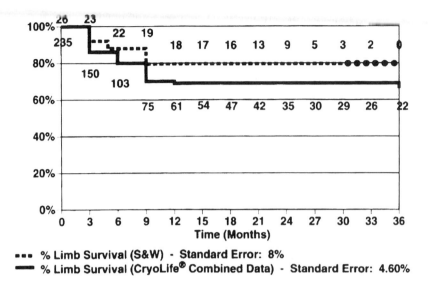

••• % Limb Survival (S&W) - Standard Error: 8%

▬▬ % Limb Survival (CryoLife® Combined Data) - Standard Error: 4.60%

FIGURE 2.

Limb salvage curves after femoral-infrapopliteal bypass grafting procedures with Cryo-Vein (CryoLife) allografts as reported by Buckley et al[16] (S & W) in their study and outlined in the CryoLife registry. *Abbreviation: S & W,* Scott & White Clinic. (Courtesy of Buckley CJ, Abernathy S, Lee SD, et al: Suggested treatment protocol for improving patency of femoral-infrapopliteal cryopreserved saphenous vein allografts. *J Vasc Surg* 32:731-738, 2000.)

because of a decreased length of stay and a minimal use of invasive monitoring.

The vendor for cryopreserved saphenous vein allografts used in most studies, CryoLife, Inc, has reported that since 1986, more than 7000 allografts have been shipped for infrainguinal bypass procedures throughout the United States. Cryolife started a volunteer registry based on accumulated clinical data obtained from 8 centers and 20 surgeons who have been frequent users of cryopreserved vein allografts for infrainguinal arterial reconstructions. According to the registry and survival analyses, between 1991 and 1998, 381 infrainguinal bypass procedures were performed with cryopreserved vein allografts for patients who had critical limb-threatening ischemia, with a primary patency rate of 22% at 4 years, and a limb salvage rate of 70% (Figs 1 and 2). The use of anticoagulation, antiplatelet therapy, and methods to assess graft patency are barely outlined in the CryoLife registry, and therefore, no conclusive evidence can be obtained about the influence of these risk factors.

Finally, vascular allografts have been promoted as the best alternative conduit for infrainguinal arterial reconstructions in infected fields when autologous veins are unsatisfactory or unavailable.[11] This is particularly important when extra-anatomic planes remote from the infected field are not feasible and direct reconstructions are necessary. Preservation of cellular integrity with modern techniques of cryopreservation may be beneficial and produce some degree of resistance to infection when combined with aggressive antibiotic therapy. Fujitani et al[11] described 8 patients in whom cryopreserved saphenous vein allografts were used in 10 infrainguinal arterial reconstructions for limb salvage with coexisting infection (mostly prosthetic graft infections). Seven allografts were patent at a mean follow-up of 9.5 months (range, 6-14 months). The authors concluded that cryopreserved veins could be used as alternative conduits, although more definitive arterial reconstruction may be necessary once infection is controlled. Similar experience has been reported with the use of cryopreserved arterial allografts in the treatment of peripheral prosthetic graft infections in Europe.[28]

CLINICAL USE OF LYOPHILIZED SAPHENOUS VEIN ALLOGRAFTS

Our previous experimental studies and the poor results with cryopreserved vascular allografts prompted us to use lyophilized saphenous vein allografts as alternative conduits for infrainguinal arterial reconstructions.[17] Lyophilized allografts had demonstrated patency and structural integrity in both the arterial and venous systems in our prior animal studies. After greater saphenous veins are harvested from cadaveric donors, the allografts undergo a freeze-drying process under vacuum that renders the tissue nonimmunogenic. Lyophilized veins are devoid of cellular elements and consist of a collagenous conduit that once reconstituted demonstrates handling characteristics similar to those of fresh veins.[18] These veins, when allografted in dogs, were seen to reendothelialize and repopulate with smooth muscle cells.[17] During the past 2 years, 4 patients have undergone femorodistal bypass grafting procedures with lyophilized saphenous veins; these patients lacked usable autologous vein for arterial reconstruction.[18] Early graft thrombosis occurred in 3 patients who required major amputations. Duplex scans for graft surveillance did not reveal previous significant abnormalities. These cases demonstrated that the clinical use of lyophilized venous allografts for infrainguinal arterial reconstructions failed to yield satisfactory patency and limb salvage. Lyophilized veins, therefore, are currently not useful alternative conduits in patients with critical ischemia and no suitable autologous vein grafts. Because lyophilized veins are readily available and inexpensive compared with other preserved veins and are easily stored, we think that further investigative studies are warranted. Our current efforts are directed to assess long-term patency, thombogenicity, and durability of endothelial-seeded lyophilized veins used as arterial conduits. Improving cellular seeding and modifying the host inflammatory response may be required before lyophilized veins can be used as effective arterial conduits. Moreover, the institution of a treatment protocol of anticoagulation may improve allograft patency of lyophilized veins. The potential use, effect, and safety of these allografts and treatment protocols should be assessed in the context of controlled clinical trials.

FUTURE DIRECTIONS

Although significant laboratory and clinical experience with venous allografts has been accumulated, further studies are still needed to find a vascular allograft that is fully biocompatible, nonthrombogenic, durable, porous enough to permit ingrowth of tissue, and suitable to maintain anastomotic integrity. Meanwhile, the role of current cryopreserved vein allografts should be investigated in the context of prospective, controlled, randomized clinical trials. In particular, studies comparing vein allografts with prosthetic grafts should be undertaken; these comparisons should also include procedures with prosthetic grafts and different types of outflow anastomoses (vein cuffs or patches and distal arteriovenous fistulas). Only better results would justify further clinical use of vascular allografts. Cryopreserved arterial allografts may also be compared with saphenous vein allografts. Moreover, the efficacy and safety of specific anticoagulation protocols to improve the results of lower extremity revascularization with vein allografts need to be assessed. If the results reported by Buckley et al[16] in their study can be reproduced in the context of a controlled, randomized clinical trial, cryopreserved vein allografts would represent an exciting alternative conduit for infrainguinal arterial reconstruction. The duration of anticoagulation also needs to be determined.

Modulating the immune response with adequate immunosuppression, particularly until repopulation of both endothelial and smooth muscle cells by host origin cells occurs, may confer better allograft patency and function, but a satisfactory regimen in human beings needs to be established. Repopulation or cellular seeding of venous allografts with host cells before implantation may decrease antigenicity and thereby significantly attenuate the host immune response. Strategies to create a nonimmunogenic allograft may obviate the need for immunosuppression. Cryopreserved vein allografts seeded with autologous endothelial cells are new tissue-engineered alternative grafts that need to be better characterized and, in particular, their utility in peripheral reconstructions should be determined.

Finally, studies from single institutions have included limited numbers of patients gathered over extended periods. Therefore, multi-institutional, randomized controlled trials are necessary, and such projects would be better served if sponsored by our specialty organizations.

CONCLUSION

Cryopreserved vein allografts have been used with variable results as alternative conduits for infrainguinal arterial reconstruction for limb salvage when suitable autologous vein is not available. Although acceptable limb salvage rates are usually obtained, cumulative patency rates continue to be suboptimal. Antigenicity and rejection are assumed to account in part for graft failure. Given the high cost and early failure rates, we recommend limited use of cryopreserved vein allografts in the context of clinical trials. Extreme circumstances that preclude the use of prosthetic grafts may be an indication for choosing cryopreserved veins. Immunosuppression has achieved partial success and is associated with significant cost and morbidity. A consistent anticoagulation protocol appears to improve allograft patency and limb salvage, although any potential benefit needs to be assessed with controlled clinical trials. The clinical use of lyophilized venous allografts for infrainguinal arterial reconstructions has failed to yield satisfactory patency and limb salvage. Lyophilized veins, therefore, are not useful alternative grafts in patients with critical ischemia and no suitable autologous vein grafts. Improving cellular seeding and modifying the host inflammatory response may be required before vein allografts can be used as effective arterial conduits.

REFERENCES

1. Kent KC, Whittemore AD, Mannick JA: Short-term and midterm results of an all-autogenous tissue policy for infrainguinal reconstruction. *J Vasc Surg* 9:107-114, 1989.
2. Veith FJ, Gupta SK, Ascer E, et al: Six-year prospective multicenter randomized comparison of autologous saphenous vein and expanded polytetrafluoroethylene grafts in infrainguinal arterial reconstructions. *J Vasc Surg* 3:104-114, 1986.

3. Woavor FA, Barlow CR, Edwards WH, et al: The lesser saphenous vein: Autogenous tissue for lower extremity revascularization. *J Vasc Surg* 5:687-692, 1987.

4. Albertini JN, Barral X, Branchereau A, et al: Long-term results of arterial allograft below-knee bypass grafts for limb salvage: A retrospective multicenter study. *J Vasc Surg* 31:426-435, 2000.

5. Lehalle B, Geschier C, Fieve G, et al: Early rupture and degeneration of cryopreserved arterial allografts. *J Vasc Surg* 25:751-752, 1997.

6. Harris RW, Schneider PA, Andros G, et al: Allograft vein bypass: Is it an acceptable alternative for infrapopliteal revascularization? *J Vasc Surg* 18:553-559, 1993.

7. Walker PJ, Mitchell RS, McFadden PM, et al: Early experience with cryopreserved saphenous vein allografts as a conduit for complex limb-salvage procedures. *J Vasc Surg* 18:561-569, 1993.

8. Shah RM, Faggioli GL, Mangione S, et al: Early results with cryopreserved saphenous vein allografts for infrainguinal bypass. *J Vasc Surg* 18:965-971, 1993.

9. Matsuura JH, Johansen KH, Rosenthal D, et al: Cryopreserved femoral vein grafts for difficult hemodialysis access. *Ann Vasc Surg* 14:50-55, 2000.

10. Dalsing MC, Raju S, Wakefield TW, et al: A multicenter, phase I evaluation of cryopreserved venous valve allografts for the treatment of chronic deep venous insufficiency. *J Vasc Surg* 30:854-864, 1999.

11. Fujitani RM, Bassiouny HS, Gewertz BL, et al: Cryopreserved saphenous vein allogenic homografts: An alternative conduit in lower extremity arterial reconstruction in infected fields. *J Vasc Surg* 15:519-526, 1992.

12. Harris L, O'brien-Irr M, Ricotta JJ: Long-term assessment of cryopreserved vein bypass grafting success. *J Vasc Surg* 33:528-532, 2001.

13. Carpenter JP, Tomaszewski JE: Immunosuppression for human saphenous vein allograft bypass surgery: A prospective randomized trial. *J Vasc Surg* 26:32-42, 1997.

14. Carpenter JP, Tomaszewski JE: Human saphenous vein allograft bypass grafts: Immune response. *J Vasc Surg* 27:492-499, 1998.

15. Posner MP, Makhoul RG, Altman M, et al: Early results of infrageniculate arterial reconstruction using cryopreserved homograft saphenous conduit (CADVEIN) and combination low-dose systemic immunosuppression. *J Am Coll Surg* 183:208-216, 1996.

16. Buckley CJ, Abernathy S, Lee SD, et al: Suggested treatment protocol for improving patency of femoral-infrapopliteal cryopreserved saphenous vein allografts. *J Vasc Surg* 32:731-738, 2000.

17. Goldman MH, Floering DA, French DR, et al: Lyophilized veins as arterial interposition grafts. *Cryobiology* 18:306-312, 1981.

18. Timaran CH, Stevens SL, Freeman MB, et al: Infrainguinal bypass grafting using lyophilized saphenous vein allografts for limb salvage. *Cardiovasc Surg* 10:315-319, 2002.

19. Wengerter K, Dardik H: Biological vascular grafts. *Semin Vasc Surg* 12: 46-51, 1999.
20. Brockbank KG, Donovan TJ, Ruby ST, et al: Functional analysis of cryo-preserved veins. Preliminary report. *J Vasc Surg* 11:94-100, 1990.
21. Johnson TR, Tomaszewski JE, Carpenter JP: Cellular repopulation of human vein allograft bypass grafts. *J Vasc Surg* 31:994-1002, 2000.
22. Benedetto B, Lipkowitz G, Madden R, et al: Use of cryopreserved cadaveric vein allograft for hemodialysis access precludes kidney transplantation because of allosensitization. *J Vasc Surg* 34:139-142, 2001.
23. Lamm P, Juchem G, Milz S, et al: Autologous endothelialized vein allograft: A solution in the search for small-caliber grafts in coronary artery bypass graft operations. *Circulation* 104:I108-I114, 2001.
24. Rutherford RB, Baker JD, Ernst C, et al: Recommended standards for reports dealing with lower extremity ischemia: Revised version. *J Vasc Surg* 26:517-538, 1997.
25. Martin RS III, Edwards WH, Mulherin JL Jr, et al: Cryopreserved saphenous vein allografts for below-knee lower extremity revascularization. *Ann Surg* 219:664-672, 1994.
26. Leseche G, Penna C, Bouttier S, et al: Femorodistal bypass using cryopreserved venous allografts for limb salvage. *Ann Vasc Surg* 11:230-236, 1997.
27. Kuang AA, Renz JF, Ferrell LD, et al: Failure patterns of cryopreserved vein grafts in liver transplantation. *Transplantation* 62:742-747, 1996.
28. Verhelst R, Lacroix V, Vraux H, et al: Use of cryopreserved arterial homografts for management of infected prosthetic grafts: A multicentric study. *Ann Vasc Surg* 14:602-607, 2000.

Part IV

Basic Science

CHAPTER 14

Strategies in Preventing Intimal Hyperplasia

Jose Roberto M. Borromeo, MD
Fellow of Vascular Surgery, Yale University School of Medicine, New Haven, Conn

Bauer E. Sumpio, MD
Professor and Chief of Vascular Surgery, Yale University School of Medicine, New Haven, Conn

Revascularization remains the standard of care for patients with significant lower extremity ischemia. Adjunctive percutaneous techniques including angioplasty and stenting have likewise become significant tools in the vascular surgeon's armamentarium in the treatment of arterial occlusive disease. Whereas significant experience with these modalities continues, failure after intervention remains a significant problem. Nearly one third of vein grafts and half of prosthetic conduits will stop functioning during the patient's life span. Although the outcomes for standard infrainguinal reconstruction have improved as surgical techniques have been refined during the past 2 decades, the long-term patency of these grafts remains a significant concern for vascular surgeons. Likewise, although graft surveillance strategies have facilitated early intervention of conduits that would otherwise have failed, graft failure requiring further revascularization interventions or, in many cases, amputation is not uncommon. More and more, increasing attention has focused on understanding the different processes involved in restenosis and subsequent graft failure.

CLINICAL IMPLICATIONS OF INTIMAL HYPERPLASIA

Significant clinical experience with various techniques of infrainguinal reconstruction has been documented in large studies. The most important factor influencing long-term patency of the vascular

conduit is the graft material.[1] Autogenous artery or vein is the pre
ferred conduit in replacing or bypassing areas of significant stenosis.
It remains the gold standard by which all conduits are compared.
Five-year patency rates for autogenous vein grafts have been reported between 60% and 80%. Infrapopliteal bypasses with autogenous vein fare less favorably than above-knee reconstructions. In
the absence of suitable vein, polytetrafluoroethylene (PTFE) has
been the most common prosthetic material used. Overall 5-year patency rates are significantly less for PTFE than for vein, and results
of PTFE grafts placed in the infrapopliteal position remain poor
(Table 1).[2]

Graft failure in the first 30 days is generally because of technical
reasons. Inherent limitations ranging from the quality of the available conduit, poor outflow, and even selection of an improper operation are the most commonly identified factors. Grafts that fail after 2
or 3 years are thought to be caused by progression of the underlying
atherosclerotic condition. Intermediate to these periods, intimal hyperplasia is the predominant process involved and occurs 60% to
80% of the time at the distal anastomosis. Much higher failure rates
are noted in longer grafts of smaller diameter where flow rates are
lower.

Significant stenosis caused by intimal hyperplasia is found in
nearly all clinical scenarios after vascular intervention. It occurs in
up to 30% of coronary arteries after angioplasty, in more than 10%
of vein grafts after peripheral bypass and in 52% to 75% of coronary
vein bypasses. Intimal hyperplasia is responsible for nearly 60% of
graft failures after peripheral arterial reconstruction.[3] Similarly, intimal hyperplasia is the predominant lesion identified in intermediate and late failure after angioplasty and stenting (Table 2). The
search for improved long-term clinical success after these interventions has led to a significant effort towards understanding the processes involved in the development of intimal hyperplasia.

TABLE 1.

Five-Year Primary Patency Rates After Infrainguinal Bypass Grafting Using
Autogenous Vein Graft and Prosthetic Grafts

Location	Vein Graft	Prosthetic Graft
Above knee popliteal	75%	38%-61%
Below knee popliteal	64%	12%-22%
Paramalleolar	40%-61%	

(Data adapted from Whittemore AD, Belkin M: Infrainguinal bypass, in Rutherford RB (ed):
Vascular Surgery, ed 5. Philadelphia, WB Saunders, 2000, pp 998-1018.)

TABLE 2.
Five-Year Primary Patency Rates After Percutaneous Transluminal Angioplasty
Alone and Angioplasty With Stent Placement

Angioplasty	
Iliac artery	34%-85%
Femoral-popliteal	26%-60%
Angioplasty and Stenting	
Iliac	63%-86%
Femoral-popliteal	39%-80%
Infrapopliteal	20%-65%

(Data adapted from Schneider PA, Rutherford RB: Endovascular interventions in the management of chronic lower extremity ischemia, in Rutherford RB (ed): *Vascular Surgery*, ed 5. Philadelphia, WB Saunders, 2000, pp 1035-1069.)

PATHOPHYSIOLOGY OF INTIMAL HYPERPLASIA

Intimal hyperplasia is an abnormal proliferative response to endothelial disruption or mural injury. Intimal hyperplasia occurs in nearly every vascular intervention. This adaptive process involves a complex interaction between the endothelial cells, macrophages, and smooth muscle cells in the media and adventitia, as well as the platelets and various cytokines activated during the normal reponse to injury. The hyperplastic response is said to correlate with the degree of injury (Fig 1).[3]

Two main theories have been proposed to explain the series of events leading to the development of intimal hyperplasia. The first involves the assumption that local hemodynamic forces play a role in the development of these lesions. When normal laminar flow is altered, such as after the creation of an anastomosis, areas of flow separation, recirculation, and stagnation result. This mechanical theory postulates that the initial stimulus for the hyperplastic response is intimal activation in response to flow dynamics. Areas of low wall shear stress result in greater intimal proliferation. In peripheral bypasses and arteriovenous access grafts, intimal hyperplasia is found to occur within the recipient artery or vein around and just beyond the anastomosis, and tends to be localized to the heel, toe, and floor.[4] In situations where endothelial disruption is not the initial insult, a chronic but nondenuding form of injury may result from various hemodynamic factors created as a consequence of the anastomosis. Physical forces such as blood flow patterns and pressure may modulate vascular structure by altering the local cellular expression of various biochemical factors secreted by the cells in the vessel wall.

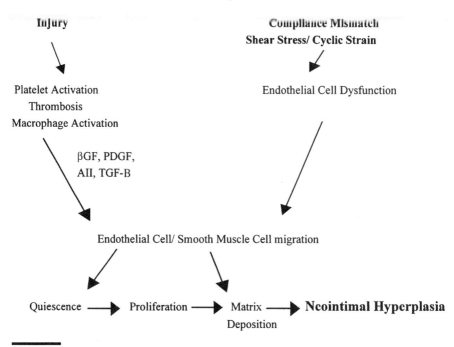

FIGURE 1.

Diagram of putative mechanisms involved in the development of intimal hyperplasia after injury. *Abbreviations: bFGF,* basic fibroblast growth factor; *PDGF,* platelet-derived growth factor; *AII,* angiotensin II; *TGF-β,* transforming growth factor-β. (Adapted from Clowes AW, Reddy MA: Prevention of stenosis after vascular reconstruction: Pharmacologic control of intimal hyperplasia: A review. *J Vasc Surg* 13: 885-891, 1991.)

A compliance mismatch between the graft and native vessel likewise may contribute further to the cellular response to these hemodynamic forces. When vein grafts are used in arterial reconstruction, their otherwise compliant nature under low pressures in the venous system is significantly reduced when subjected to constant arterial pressures. The resulting relative stiffness of the vein graft results in almost no change in caliber during the various ranges of arterial pressure. A significant compliance mismatch between the vein graft and native artery results. Prosthetic grafts exhibit considerable compliance mismatch, and this property is thought to result in the different patency rates of these grafts. Alterations in hemodynamic forces at the various portions of the distal anastomosis correlate with the locations where intimal hyperplasia most commonly occurs.[5-7]

The biological theory proposes that certain cellular or noncellular components in the circulation interact with the vascular conduit and trigger a cellular response in the recipient artery.

After angioplasty or endarterectomy, endothelial cell disruption leads to platelet aggregation and thrombosis. In these clinical scenarios, subsequent platelet activation and degranulation result in the release of various vasoactive and thrombotic factors, as well as cytokines and growth factors. Among them, platelet-derived growth factor and basic fibroblast growth factor are among the most important. They are potent activators and chemoattractants for smooth muscle cells and myofibroblasts. Macrophages have also been postulated to be important modulators of the reponse to injury phenomenon. As a result, smooth muscle cells from the media migrate to the intima and eventually undergo rapid proliferation. Migration occurs within several hours, and the proliferative response begins as early as the first 24 hours. Subsequent matrix deposition results in significant intimal thickening and luminal narrowing that continues over indefinite periods.[1]

GENERAL STRATEGIES IN PREVENTING INTIMAL HYPERPLASIA

Mechanical and biological strategies are used to prevent intimal hyperplasia. They are outlined in Table 3 and discussed below.

TABLE 3.
General Strategies in Preventing Intimal Hyperplasia

I. Mechanical Strategies
    A. Alteration of hemodynamic forces
    B. Changing the geometry of the anastomosis
II. Biological Strategies
    A. Inhibition of SMC Migration and Proliferation
        1. Pharmacologic
            a. Antiplatelet agents
            b. Anticoagulation
        2. Brachytherapy
        3. Gene Therapy
            a. VEGF
            b. E2F decoy
            c. Nitric oxide synthase
        4. Local Drug Delivery
            a. Actinomycin D
            b. Taxol
            c. Sirolimus/Rapamycin

Abbreviations: SMC, Smooth muscle cell; *VEGF,* vascular endothelial growth factor; *E2F,* E2F transcription factor.

MECHANICAL STRATEGIES

Intimal hyperplasia is the single most important factor affecting long-term graft patency. It results in critical graft stenosis and is associated with an overall reduction in graft flow, leading to subsequent graft thrombosis. Hemodynamic factors play a significant role in the development of intimal hyperplasia after arterial bypass. These factors have been shown experimentally in hemodynamic flow models simulating various end-to-side graft configurations.[4-6]

Arteries are described to be anisotropic. They exhibit a nonlinear degree of radial deformation in relation to increased intraluminal pressure. The initial stress is borne by the elastin, and later by less elastic collagen fibers at higher pressures. Vein grafts have significantly fewer smooth muscle cells and elastin fibers than do arteries. Although anisotropic, they are relatively incompliant when exposed to higher mean pressures in the arterial circulation. Similarly, prosthetic grafts including PTFE and Dacron exhibit significant stiffness and lower compliance at varying mean pressure ranges. Mismatch in the elastic or compliance properties between the graft and recipient artery has been implicated in the etiology of intimal hyperplasia at anastomotic sites.[7] Disparity in the compliance at this junction has been postulated to cause smooth muscle cell activation when exposed to anomalous cyclic strain forces and mitogens released by platelets activated by disturbances in flow patterns.

Recently, Tai et al[7] described the development of a prosthetic graft in which compliant polycarbonate polyurethane was used. They demonstrated that the compliant polycarbonate polyurethane graft was a better compliance and stiffness match to artery than vein grafts and other prosthetic grafts. This graft is currently undergoing clinical evaluation as a potential conduit for infrainguinal bypass procedures.

The concept of changing the geometry at the distal anastomosis stems from studies demonstrating that optimization of flow patterns at the anastomosis may prevent progression of intimal hyperplasia. Strong experimental evidence illustrates that areas involving the heel, toe, and floor of the anastomosis, where lesions of intimal hyperplasia occur, correspond to regions of flow separation and low wall shear stress. Primary alterations in flow as a result of various anastomotic cuff techniques (Fig 2) affect wall shear stress. The vortex patterns demonstrated by using prosthetic grafts with a Miller vein cuff as well as a precuffed PTFE graft (Distaflo, Impra) result in persistent vortex patterns throughout the cardiac cycle.[5] This leads to a continued washout effect over the entire cuff cavity and possibly enhanced mixing of blood components. The corresponding de-

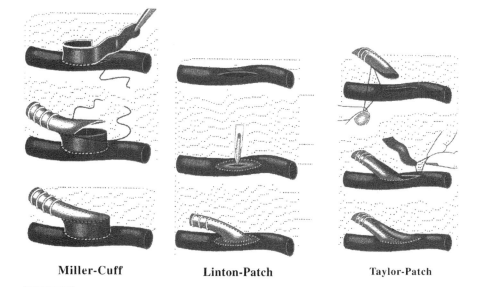

Miller-Cuff   **Linton-Patch**   **Taylor-Patch**

FIGURE 2.

Distal anastomotic techniques. (Courtesy of Noori N, Scherer R, Perktold K, et al: Blood flow in distal end-to-side anastomoses with PTFE and a venous patch: Results of an in vitro flow visualization study. *Eur J Vasc Endovasc Surg* 18:191-200. Copyright 2001, by permission of the publisher WB Saunders Company Limited, London.)

crease in relative regions of stasis are thought to minimize the effects of processes involved in the development of intimal hyperplasia.[6]

The results of various anastomotic techniques are illustrated in Table 4.

BIOLOGICAL STRATEGIES
Antiplatelet Agents and Anticoagulation

Antiplatelet and anticoagulant agents have been in clinical use as adjuncts in enhancing graft patency for several decades. Aspirin exerts its effect on platelet aggregation by irreversibly inactivating the cyclooxygenase activity of prostaglandin synthase. Although it has been demonstrated to reduce periprocedure thrombosis, it has no impact on vessel restenosis. The thienopyridines (clopidogrel and ticlopidine) have been shown to block platelet activation more effectively by their inhibition of adenosine diphosphate (ADP)-related platelet aggregation. The final common pathway of platelet activation lies in the glycoprotein IIb/IIIa receptor level. Recently, specific inhibitors to these receptors, such as abciximab (Reopro), have been demonstrated to have significant effects on decreasing the incidence of major adverse cardiac events.[8]

The rationale for use of these agents has been to prevent early thrombosis and occlusion related to platelet aggregation, which can later contribute to the development of intimal hyperplasia. Experimental evidence, however, in the latter situation has been variable. It appears that platelet aggregation is not the sole process involved in such lesions, and so most platelet inhibitors may not significantly attenuate the progression of intimal hyperplasia. Inhibitors of platelet glycoprotein IIb/IIIa, however, may also inhibit smooth muscle cell proliferation, but this has not been demonstrated consistently in clinical trials.[8]

Brachytherapy

Radiotherapy has been used extensively to inhibit both benign and malignant cellular proliferative lesions. Its use in preventing restenosis is based on the inhibition of smooth muscle cell proliferation. The energy from the radioactive isotope results in double-stranded DNA breaks and subsequent block in cell division.[9]

Experimental evidence regarding the use of both external beam irradiation and endoluminal delivery has been described in animal and, more recently, in human studies. There has been significant concern as to the safety of vascular irradiation in light of variable dosage windows noted in the different studies. In high doses, vascular injury may result, leading to subsequent fibrosis and occlusion.

TABLE 4.
Primary Patency Rates Using Various Distal Anastomotic Techniques

Type	Author	Patency Years	Primary Patency Rates
Above Knee Popliteal			
Taylor Patch	Taylor	5	77%
Miller Cuff	Raptis	3	69%
Miller Cuff	Stonebridge	2	72%
Below Knee Popliteal			
Linton Patch	Batson	4	65%
Taylor Patch	Taylor	5	65%
Miller Cuff	Raptis	3	57%
Miller Cuff	Pappas	2	75%
Infrapopliteal			
Taylor Patch	Taylor	5	54%
Miller Cuff	Pappas	2	62%

(Adapted from Steinthorsson G, Sumpio B: Clinical and biological relevance of vein cuff anastomosis. *Acta Chir Belg* 99:282-288, 1999. Used with permission.)

There is considerable evidence in animal studies of coronary, carotid, and iliac artery models of injury followed by radiation treatment, that radiation reduces perivascular fibrosis and intimal hyperplasia.[10] Most of the experience in human beings is derived from clinical trials after coronary artery intervention.

Several randomized trials reported encouraging data in preventing coronary restenosis. The GAMMA I trial involved 252 patients with long-segment coronary in-stent restenosis treated with catheter-based delivery. This study demonstrated a reduction in the rate of repeated revascularization from 46% to 31% at 9 months. The START trial involving 472 patients, and the INHIBIT trial with 332 patients revealed a reduction in the need for reintervention, from 24% to 16% in the START trial and from 31% to 20% in the INHIBIT trial, at 9-month follow-up.

A study in Europe demonstrated an increased cumulative patency after superficial femoral artery angioplasty in 113 randomized patients. The radiation treatment group had a patency rate of 63.6% versus 35.3% in the control group at 1-year follow-up.[9] The SCRIPPS trial published in 1997 described significantly improved 1-year event-free survival in patients receiving intraluminal irradiation after coronary angioplasty and stenting. This correlated with findings on follow-up angiography and intravascular ultrasound.[9]

Recent trials have reported on the use of radioactive coronary stents. Albeiro et al[10] reported their experience with the beta-emitting Isostent (Isotent, San Carlos, Calif) of varying doses of radiation. Their findings illustrate a significant reduction of in-stent restenosis from intimal hypeplasia, most notably with the stents with higher radiation doses.

Multiple studies, however, noted significant concerns regarding the safety of radiotherapy for restenosis. One concern is the finding of late thrombosis in 3% to 10% of patients, irrespective of the isotope and delivery system tested.[10] Another phenomenon observed by numerous investigators is the development of edge restenosis beyond the stent or delivery area. This is thought to be caused by a drop-off effect in radiation dose at these segments, and irradiation at low doses has been demonstrated to stimulate neointimal hyperplasia. Although there is considerable potential benefit of this modality, significant concerns remain about the ideal conditions and doses for widespread clinical application.

Gene Therapy

The increasing understanding of the molecular biology of vascular cell activation and proliferation has allowed the use of various tech-

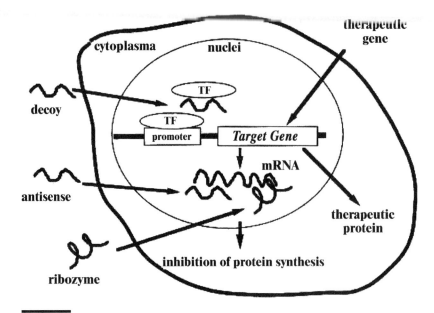

FIGURE 3.

Strategies to prevent restenosis. (Courtesy of Morishita R, Aoki M, Kaneda Y, et al: Gene therapy in vascular medicine: Recent advances and future perspectives. *Pharmacol Ther* 91:105-114, 2001. Used with permission.)

niques at the gene expression level. Gene therapy involves the introduction of normal genes into somatic cells to correct underlying conditions by inducing the synthesis of specific gene products in vivo. Among the various techniques available, gene augmentation is most commonly used in the treatment of vascular diseases. Induction of angiogenesis in patients with nonreconstructable arterial occlusive disease is one application of such methods.

Multiple approaches towards altering the cellular response by using various gene products have been described in animal models and in small clinical studies. Recent application of DNA technology has provided new techniques to inhibit specific gene expression (Fig 3). The use of special RNA sequences known as ribozymes that can cleave specific target mRNA molecules has been proposed. Another method involves the use of antisense oligodeoxynucleotides, which inhibit mRNA translation by binding to specific mRNA sequences. Lastly, the more stable double-stranded DNA sequences with high affinity for specific target transcription factors are used as "decoy" sequences. The resultant binding of the DNA to the transcription factor alters gene expression (Fig 3).[11] Recent investigations have focused mainly on the use of these gene products by gene transfer and expression in target vascular lesions. Among the numerous potential gene candidates, significant research has been undertaken with vascular endothelial growth factor (VEGF), nitric oxide synthase (NOS), and the antisense oligodeoxynucleotide E2F decoy.

VEGF.—The processes responsible for the development of intimal hyperplastic lesions involve complex cellular interactions. The role of endothelial cells in these processes has yet to to be fully understood. It has been postulated that rapid regeneration of these endothelial cells after injury may modulate vascular growth via endothelial-derived antiproliferative cytokines. Asahara and his group reported significant inhibition of neointimal formation by VEGF transfer.[11]

Clinical research of therapeutic angiogenesis using VEGF gene transfer was pioneered by Isner's laboratory in 1994. By using naked $VEGF_{165}$ plasmid injected intramuscularly in patients with critical limb ischemia, they demonstrated clinical improvement in a small group of patients. This correlated with increased collateral formation demonstrated by angiography and later, magnetic resonance angiography.[11] Further trials in patients with coronary ischemia that used different angiogenic factors, including VEGF-2, and $VEGF_{121}$, and various delivery techniques have been reported. Although certain studies demonstrated an objective increase in myocardial blood flow, clinical outcomes were variable and ranged from decreased nitroglycerin requirements to subjective improvement in overall functional status.[11]

These trials, even in a small number of patients, demonstrate significant potential application of angiogenic gene therapy for critical ischemia in patients with severe, nonreconstructible coronary and peripheral arterial disease.

E2F DECOY.—The process of smooth muscle cell proliferation is dependent on the coordinated activation of a series of cell-cycle regulatory genes. The critical element of the cycle progression involves the formation of the E2F cyclin A/cyclin-dependent kinase-2 (cdk2) complex (Fig 4). This E2F-1 transcription factor is released from a regulatory complex involving the hyperphosphorylation of the retinoblastoma (Rb) gene product at late G1 phase. The resulting free E2F has been associated with upregulated expression of a dozen genes involved in DNA synthesis and cell-cycle progression, resulting in cellular proliferation.[12] Morishita et al[11] demonstrated that successful transfection of E2F decoy into rat vascular smooth muscle cells effectively bound the dissociated E2F. Bound E2F was unable to transactivate the essential cell-cycle regulatory proteins, thereby inhibiting smooth muscle cell proliferation and intimal hyperplasia. Dzau and his team demonstrated successful inhibition of the upregulation process in vascular cells by blocking this transcription factor with double-stranded decoy oligodeoxynucleotide bearing the E2F binding site.[12] The single-center PREVENT trial by Mann et al[13] was a prospective randomized trial in which E2F decoy was delivered ex vivo in 17 patients undergoing lower extremity vein bypass grafting. At 12 months, fewer graft occlusions and stenoses were noted in the treatment group.

Preliminary results of the PREVENT II trial have recently been presented. This randomized, double-blind, controlled phase 2b study involved 200 patients who underwent nonelective coronary bypass surgery and were randomly assigned to either E2F decoy or

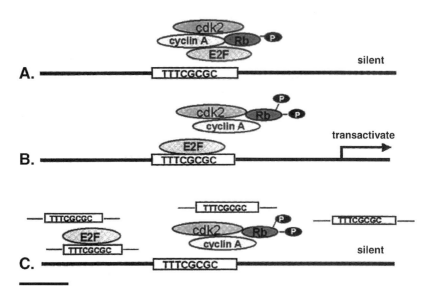

FIGURE 4.

Principles of E2F decoy strategy. **A,** In a quiescent cell state, the transcription factor E2F is complexed with retinoblastoma gene product *(Rb),* cyclin A, and cyclin-dependent kinase-2 *(ckd2).* **B,** Hyperphosphorylation of retinoblastoma gene product releases free E2F, which binds to enhancer regions of cell-cycle regulatory genes, resulting in their transactivation. **C,** The E2F decoy double-stranded oligodeoxynucleotide binds to free E2F, preventing E2F-mediated transactivation of cell-cycle regulatory genes. (Courtesy of Ehsan A, Mann M, Dell'Acqua G, et al: Long-term stabilization of vein graft wall architecture and prolonged resistance to experimental atherosclerosis after E2F decoy oligonucleotide therapy. *J Thorac Cardiovasc Surg* 121:714-722, 2001. Used with permission.)

TABLE 5.
Effects of Nitric Oxide on the Vascular System

Regulation of vascular tone/Vasodilatation
Inhibits platelet aggregation and adhesion
Inhibits platelet activation
Inhibits smooth muscle cell proliferation and migration
Inhibits matrix synthesis
Reduces monocyte and neutrophil activation and chemotaxis
Reduces vascular inflammation
Antioxidant

placebo treatment. At 1-year follow-up, there was no significant difference in primary end points, defined as adverse outcomes resulting in death, myocardial infarction, or requiring reintervention. Secondary end points were assessed by angiography and intravascular ultrasound. Graft failure was detected in 27% of treated patients compared with 38% in the control group (P = .03). Vascular wall volume was reduced in the E2F decoy group on intravascular ultrasound evaluation in a subgroup of 65 patients. This study demonstrated the safety and feasibility of the E2F decoy in the prevention of vein graft stenosis after coronary revascularization.[14]

Nitric Oxide.—Nitric oxide (NO) functions as both a signaling molecule in endothelial and nerve cells and as a killer molecule in activated immune cells. NO also has significant effects on vascular cells and vasomotor tone. It mediates vasorelaxation, inhibits vascular smooth muscle cell migration and proliferation, and reduces platelet activation and vascular inflammation (Table 5). Various disease states, including hypertension, diabetes, and even atherosclerotic lesions, demonstrate reduced NO bioactivity because of either increased catabolism or decreased NO production. It is thought that impaired NO activity in the vessel wall leads to dysregulation of cell growth, migration, and matrix deposition, leading to pathologic vascular remodeling.[15]

Experimental evidence from gene transfer studies suggests that NO inhibits smooth muscle cell proliferation. Current studies focus on the potential beneficial effects of NO restoration, NO overexpression, or both, as a potential therapeutic modality in the treatment of various cardiovascular diseases, including coronary vasospasm, thrombosis, and peripheral arterial occlusive conditions.[15,16]

Studies on porcine peripheral and coronary arteries after stent-induced vascular injury by von der Leyen and Dzau[15] demonstrated inhibition of stent-induced lesions by up to 50% with the use of liposome-mediated gene transfer of inducible nitric oxide synthase (iNOS). Cable and his colleagues successfully transfected human saphenous veins with adenovirus vector encoding bovine eNOS and demonstrated functional expression of the recombinant NOS.[16] Diffusible NO is likewise thought to exert additional therapeutic potential via a paracrine effect.

The potential benefit of NO in the treatment of numerous cardiovascular diseases, including proliferative lesions such as intimal hyperplasia, has stirred considerable interest in this modality. Currently, clinical studies to determine the potential benefit and safety profiles in human subjects are under way.

Local Drug Delivery

New approaches to minimize intimal hyperplasia involve pharmacologic modulation of the local vascular biology. Previously, local concentrations of various agents could not be achieved without administering large doses, with the potential for significant systemic toxicity. By using specially coated stents and various delivery vehicles that allow for variable release of the drug, it has become possible to deliver these agents to specific target areas where restenosis in the injured vessels occur. Clinical trials with different techniques of stent coating, and various agents, such as antiproliferative drugs, immunusuppressants, and collagen inhibitors, are now under investigation (Table 6). In the following section, we describe 3 agents that are undergoing numerous clinical trials to assess their efficacy in the

TABLE 6.
Potential Candidates for Drug Elution

Antineoplastic	**Collagen Synthase Inhibitors**
Paclitaxel (Taxol)	Metalloproteinase inhibitor
Taxol derivative QP-2	Halofuginone
Vincristine	
Antithrombins	**Angiopeptin V**
Hirudin and Iloprost	
Heparin	
Immunosuppressants	**VEGF**
Sirolimus	
Tranilast	
Dexamethasone	
Tacrolimus (FK 506)	

Abbreviation: VEGF, Vascular endothelial growth factor.
(Courtesy of Regar E, Sianos G, Seruys PW: Stent development and local drug delivery. *Br Med Bull* 59:227-248, 2001. Used with permission.)

prevention of stenosis caused by intimal hyperplasia in target coronary lesions.

ACTINOMYCIN **D.**—Actinomycin D is an antibiotic with antiprolifierative properties used in the treatment of numerous malignancies, including Wilms' tumor and soft tissue sarcomas. It forms a stable complex with double-stranded DNA and subsequently inhibits DNA-primed RNA synthesis. Current studies are under way including the ACTION trial, which is using the Multi-link Tetra-D system (Guidant, Temecula, Calif) for de novo coronary lesions and restenosis with a target of 360 patients.[17]

PACLITAXEL (TAXOL).—Paclitaxel is a potent antineoplastic agent commonly used in the treatment of breast and ovarian cancer. It exerts its action on microtubule assembly through the formation of stable components and subsequent inhibition of proliferation and migration, as well as signal transduction. It has been demonstrated experimentally to inhibit smooth muscle cell proliferation in a dose-dependent manner.

Several studies have been performed for coronary lesions and include the TAXUS I trial. Sixty-one patients were randomly assigned to receive either paclitaxel-treated or control stents. The paclitaxel group demonstrated no restenosis at 6 months compared with 11% in the bare-stent group. Similarly, the late lumen loss was significantly lower in the treatment group, and cardiac-associated morbidity at 3 months was lower in the treatment group.[17] The double-blind, randomized ASPECT trial involving 177 patients demonstrated a significant dose-response inhibition of restenosis at 6-month follow-up as well, with the use of high- and low-dose Supra G (Cook/Guidant) stents (4%, 12%, and 27% stenosis with the high-dose, low-dose, and control devices, respectively).[17] Various larger studies including the TAXUS I to IV trials are under way worldwide looking at various conditions, including de novo and recurrent lesions, in multicenter large-scale trials.

RAPAMYCIN/SIROLIMUS.—Rapamycin is a naturally occurring macrolide antibiotic produced as a fermentation product of *Streptomyces hygroscopicus*. Although initially discovered in 1965 and described for its antifungal properties, the drug has only been in extensive use since 1999 for immunosuppression after renal transplantation. It has been demonstrated to have significant effects in conditions involving accelerated arteriopathy with the potential for use in various disease states, including autoimmune conditions, and in preventing coronary stenosis after cardiac transplantation.[18]

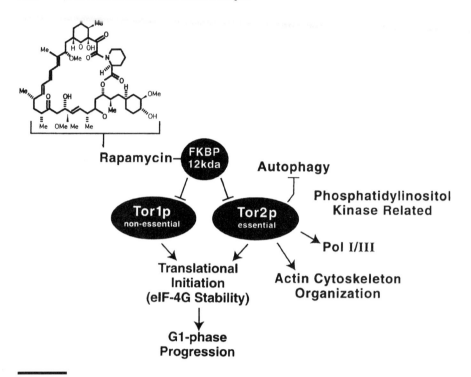

FIGURE 5.

Structure of rapamycin, the molecule with which it interacts, and the pathways which respond to its addition to cells. *Arrows* and *bars* indicate positive and negative regulation, respectively. (Courtesy of TG Cooper: Transmitting the signal of excess nitrogen in Saccharomyces cerevisiae from the Tor proteins to the GATA factors: Connecting the dots. *FEMS Microbiol Rev* 26:223-238, 2002.)

The cellular actions of rapamycin are mediated by binding to a specific intracellular immunophilin receptor protein (FKBP12) (Fig 5). Its immunosuppressive activity is mediated by inhibiting the kinase mTOR target protein, which is an important component in a pathway that regulates cell-cycle progression. In vivo and in vitro studies demonstrate blocking of the cell cycle in smooth muscle cells at the G1/S transition. mTOR inhibition also results in diminished cytokine-driven T-cell proliferation.[18]

Nonrandomized clinical studies with rapamycin-coated Velocity Bx stents (Cordis, Warren, NJ) demonstrated no significant in-stent or edge restenosis on angiographic and intravascular ultrasound evaluation during follow-up at 4, 6, and 12 months. The randomized RAVEL study involved 238 patients with similar stents. At 6-month follow-up, there was no restenosis and no loss of minimal luminal diameter in the treatment group compared with a 26.2% restenosis rate in patients who received the noncoated stent. Both groups had no reported thrombosis, but the treatment group had a 96.5% event-free survival rate compared with 72.9% in the control group.[17]

Currently, large-scale trials, including the prospective randomized SIRIUS study involving 1100 patients in 55 centers in the United States, are under way looking at 9-month and long-term clinical outcomes with sirolimus-coated stents for coronary lesions.

CONCLUSIONS

Vascular reconstruction and intervention currently remain the mainstay of treatment of arterial occlusive disease. Despite numerous advances in surgical technique and percutaneous methods, significant long-term and intermediate failure of these interventions is caused by progression of the underlying disease states and by proliferative lesions in the reparative processes involved in vascular remodeling. The prevention of intimal hyperplasia remains the most important factor in the success of such interventions. Important investigations in understanding the various processes involved in the development of intimal hyperplasia have been undertaken in recent years. Understanding these complex processes opens the door to new modalities in the treatment of these proliferative lesions.

Mechanical techniques, such as improving and optimizing hemodynamic forces with various anastomotic methods and precuffed grafts, have been used for many years with varying degrees of success. Although studies with peripheral vascular disease lags behind the experience in coronary intervention, new modalities including local drug delivery, gene therapy, and pharmacologic therapy may have significant potential benefit in minimizing these lesions and possibly increase long-term patency after arterial reconstruction.

REFERENCES

1. Steinthorsson G, Sumpio B: Clinical and biological relevance of vein cuff anastomosis. *Acta Chir Belg* 99:282-288, 1999.
2. Whittemore AD, Belkin M: Infrainguinal bypass, in Rutherford RB (ed): *Vascular Surgery*, ed 5. Philadelphia, WB Saunders, 2000, pp 998-1018.
3. Clowes AW: Pathologic intimal hyperplasia as a response to vascular injury and reconstruction, in Rutherford RB (ed): *Vascular Surgery*, ed 5. Philadelphia, WB Saunders, 2000, pp 408-418.
4. Fisher RK, How TV, Toonder IM, et al: Harnessing haemodynamic forces for the suppression of anastomotic intimal hyperplasia: The rationale for precuffed grafts. *Eur J Vasc Endovasc Surg* 21:520-528, 2001.

5. Noori N, Schoror R, Perktold K, et al: Blood flow in distal end-to-side anastomoses with PTFE and a venous patch: Results of an in vitro flow visualization study. *Eur J Vasc Endovasc Surg* 18:191-200, 2001.

6. Fisher RK, How TV, Carpenter T, et al: Optimizing Miller cuff dimensions: The influence of geometry on anastomotic flow patterns. *Eur J Vasc Endovasc Surg* 21:251-260, 2001.

7. Tai NR, Salcinski HJ, Edwards A, et al: Compliance properties of conduits used in vascular reconstructions. *Br J Surg* 87:1516-1524, 2000.

8. Harding SA, Walters DL, Palacios IF, et al: Adjunctive pharmacotherapy for coronary stenting. *Curr Opin Cardiol* 16:293-299, 2001.

9. Teirstein PS, Kuntz RE: New frontiers in interventional cardiology intravascular radiation to prevent restenosis. *Circulation* 104:2620-2626, 2001.

10. Albeiro R, Nishida T, Adamanian M, et al: Edge restenosis after implantation of high activity (32)P radioactive beta emitting stents. *Circulation* 101:2454-2457, 2000.

11. Morishita R, Aoki M, Kaneda Y, et al: Gene therapy in vascular medicine: Recent advances and future perspectives. *Pharmacol Ther* 91:105-114, 2001.

12. Ehsan A, Mann M, Dell'Acqua G, et al: Long-term stabilization of vein graft wall architecture and prolonged resistance to experimental athcrosclerosis after E2F decoy oligonucleotide therapy. *J Thorac Cardiovasc Surg* 121:714-722, 2001.

13. Mann M, Whittemore AD, Donaldson MC, et al: Ex-vivo gene therapy of human vascular bypass grafts with E2F decoy: The PREVENT single-center, randomized, controlled trial. *Lancet* 354:1493-1498, 1999.

14. Kandzari DE, Kay J, O'Shea JC, et al: Highlights from the American Heart Association Annual Scientific Sessions 2001: November 11 to 14, 2001. *Am Heart J* 143:217-224, 2002.

15. von der Leyen HE, Dzau VJ: Therapeutic potential of nitric oxide synthase gene manipulation. *Circulation* 103:2760-2765, 2001.

16. Channon KM, Qian HS, George SE: Nitric oxide synthase in atherosclerosis and vascular injury. *Arterioscler Thromb Vasc Biol* 20:1873-1881, 2000.

17. Regar E, Sianos G, Seruys PW: Stent development and local drug delivery. *Br Med Bull* 59:227-248, 2001.

18. Marx SO, Marks AR: Bench to bedside: The development of rapamycin and its applications to stent restenosis. *Circulation* 104:852-855, 2001.

Index

Nitinol frame, after endovascular
repair of abdominal aortic
aneurysms, 112

G

Gadolinium
-enhanced angiography, CT or MR,
for renal artery stenosis, 139,
148
-enhanced CT for aortic pathology,
137
-enhanced MRI before AneuRx
stent graft placement, 80
Gamma radiation, for in-stent carotid
restenosis, 3
Gantry angle simulation, in
intraoperative imaging
for endovascular interventions,
148-150
Gene
therapy in prevention of intimal
hyperplasia, 209-214
VEGF, transfer in prevention of
intimal hyperplasia, 211
Graft
bypass
coronary artery, with
simultaneous bilateral carotid
endarterectomy (*see*
Endarterectomy, carotid,
simultaneous bilateral)
to dorsalis pedis artery (*see*
Dorsalis pedis, bypass)
prosthetic
infrainguinal bypass with, 5-year
patency rates, 202
using polycarbonate polyurethane
in prevention of intimal
hyperplasia, 206
stent (*see* Stent-graft)
vein, autogenous, infrainguinal
bypass with, 5-year patency
rates, 202
Growth factor, vascular endothelial,
gene transfer, in prevention of
intimal hyperplasia, 212

H

Hardware, for imaging of aortic
pathology, 136-138
Hemobahn stent-grafts, 129-130
Hemodialysis access, cryopreserved
saphenous vein grafts for, 187
Hemodynamic forces, changes in, in
prevention of intimal
hyperplasia, 206
Heparin, in carotid stenting, 21
Horner syndrome, during carotid
body tumor surgery, 54
Hyperplasia, intimal (*see* Intimal
hyperplasia)
Hypogastric artery embolization, and
endovascular repair of
abdominal aortic aneurysms,
110, 111
Hypoxia, chronic, exposure to, and
carotid body tumors, 46

I

Iliac artery aneurysm (*see* Aneurysm,
iliac)
Imaging
in aortic aneurysm repair,
endovascular, 143-151
intraoperative, 148-150
postoperative, 150-151
preoperative, 143-148
preoperative, adjunctive studies,
148
in aortic aneurysm repair, open,
139-143
complex, 142
simple, 139-142
for aortic pathology, 135-154
hardware, 136-138
thoracic, 142-143
in carotid body tumors, 48-49
indium-111 pentetreotide, in
carotid body tumors, 49
iodine-131
metaiodobenzylguanidine, in
carotid body tumors, 48
magnetic resonance (*see* Magnetic
resonance imaging)

Information and insights you won't find anywhere else—straight from the experts!

YES! Please start my subscription to the *Advances* checked below with the current volume according to the terms described below.* I understand that I will have 30 days to examine each annual edition.

Please Print:

Name _____

Address _____

City _____ State _____ ZIP _____

Method of Payment

❑ Check (payable to **Mosby**; add the applicable sales tax for your area)

❑ VISA   ❑ MasterCard   ❑ AmEx   ❑ Bill me

Card number _____ Exp. date _____

Signature _____

❑ **Advances in Anesthesia® (YAAN)**
   $98.00 (Avail. December)

❑ **Advances in Dermatology® (YADR)**
   $98.00 (Avail. November)

❑ **Advances in Pediatrics® (YAPD)**
   $89.00 (Avail. July)

❑ **Advances in Surgery® (YASU)**
   $89.00 (Avail. September)

❑ **Advances in Vascular Surgery® (YAVS)**
   $98.00 (Avail. October)

Your Advances service guarantee:

When you subscribe to an *Advances*, you will receive notice of future annual volumes about two months before publication. To receive the new edition, do nothing—we'll send you the new volume as soon as it is available. (Applicable sales tax is added to each shipment.) If you want to discontinue, the advance notice allows you time to notify us of your decision. If you are not completely satisfied, you have 30 days to return any *Advances*.

BUSINESS REPLY MAIL

FIRST-CLASS MAIL   PERMIT NO 7135   ORLANDO FL

POSTAGE WILL BE PAID BY ADDRESSEE

PERIODICALS ORDER FULFILLMENT DEPT
MOSBY
ELSEVIER SCIENCE
6277 SEA HARBOR DR
ORLANDO FL 32821-9852

VISIT OUR HOME PAGE!
www.mosby.com/periodicals

Mosby
A Division of Elsevier Science

11830 Westline Industrial Drive
St. Louis, MO   63146 U.S.A.